A DAY IN THE LIFE OF A
Medical Detective

by Adam Carter
Photography by Bob Duncan

Troll Associates

Library of Congress Cataloging in Publication Data

Carter, Adam.
  A day in the life of a medical detective.

  Summary: Follows an epidemiologist through a day at work at the Centers for Disease Control in Atlanta, Georgia.
      1. Epidemiologists—Juvenile literature.   2. Epidemiology—Vocational guidance—Juvenile literature.
  3. Richards, Rick—Juvenile literature.   4. Epidemiologists—United States—Juvenile literature.   5. Centers for Disease Control (U.S.)—Juvenile literature.
  [1. Richards, Rick.   2. Epidemiologists.   3. Centers for Disease Control (U.S.)   4. Occupations]   I. Duncan, Bob (Bob L.), ill.   II. Title.
  RA653.5.C37   1985   614.4'092'4   84-8851
  ISBN 0-8167-0097-4 (lib. bdg.)
  ISBN 0-8167-0098-2 (pbk.)

Copyright © 1985 by Troll Associates, Mahwah, New Jersey.
All rights reserved. No part of this book may be used or reproduced in any manner whatsoever without written permission from the publisher.
Printed in the United States of America.

10 9 8 7 6 5 4 3 2 1

The author and publisher wish to thank Dr. Rick Richards, Dr. Nancy Lee, Dr. Ward Cates, Dwan Hightower, Cornelia McGrath, Tony Sanchez, and especially Sandy Ford for their generous cooperation and assistance.

Dr. Rick Richards hurries to a weekly seminar at the Centers for Disease Control—CDC, for short—in Atlanta, Georgia. Dr. Richards is a "medical detective" who specializes in controlling epidemics. He tries to identify contagious diseases and stop them before they can spread through an entire town, county, or state.

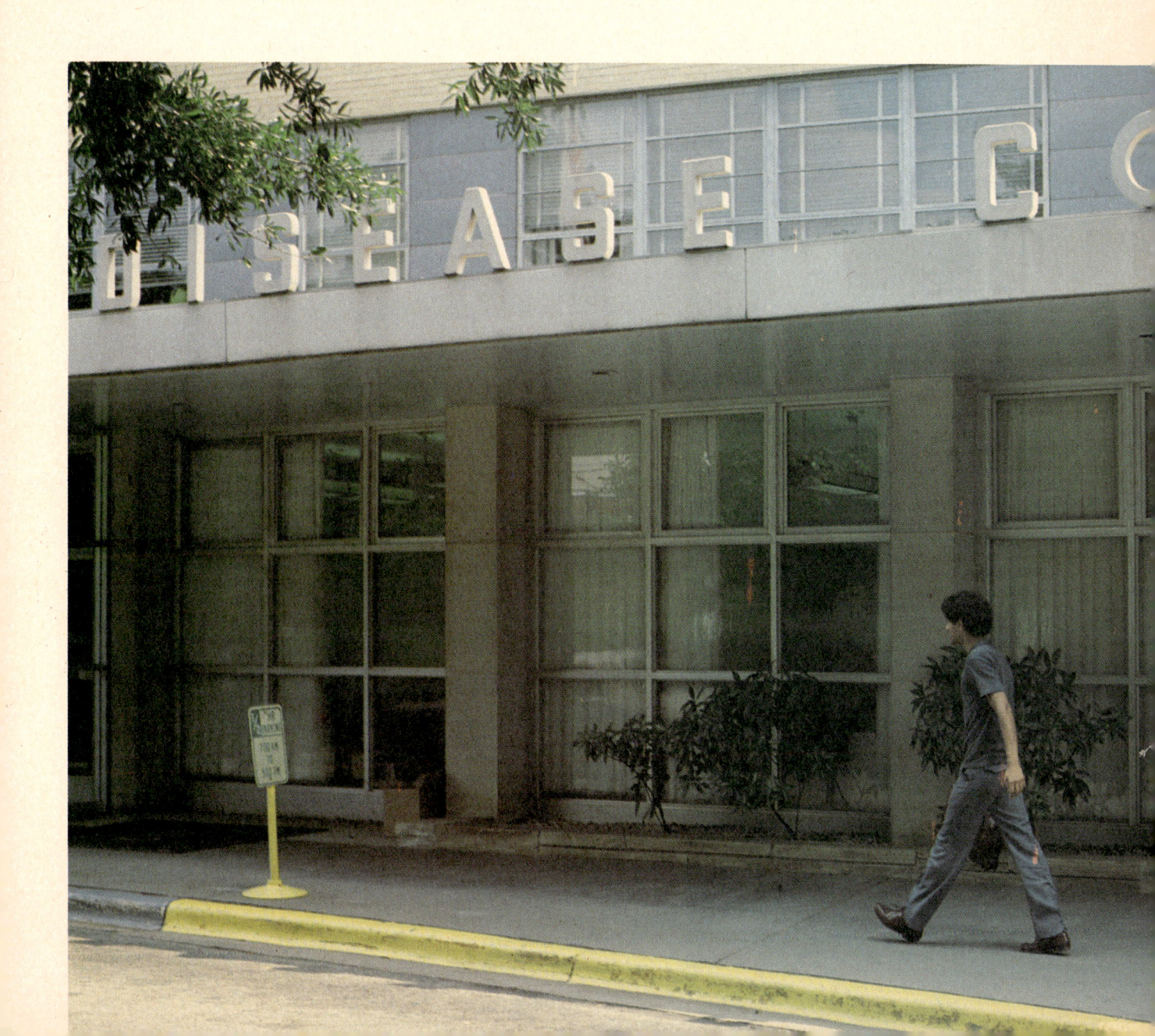

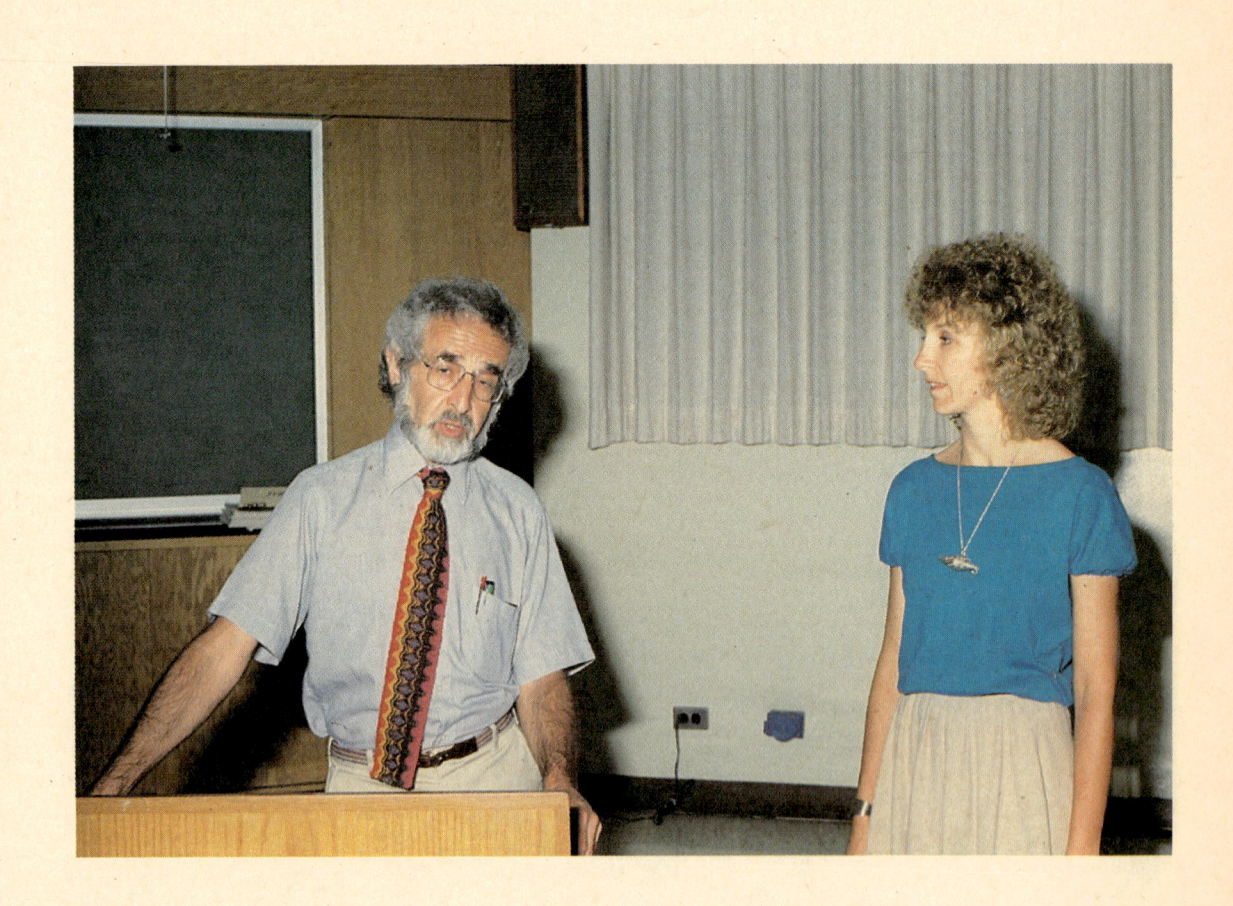

At the seminar, members of the CDC medical staff discuss diseases they are investigating. Dr. Richards arrives just as the first speaker is being introduced. She is Dr. Nancy Lee—a medical detective who has been working on an epidemic that is spreading through many villages in Africa.

Dr. Lee brings the group up to date on her investigation, and shows slides of an African village threatened by the disease. She explains the steps CDC has recommended to halt the epidemic. Dr. Lee's report will be released as a warning to people who plan to travel to the area.

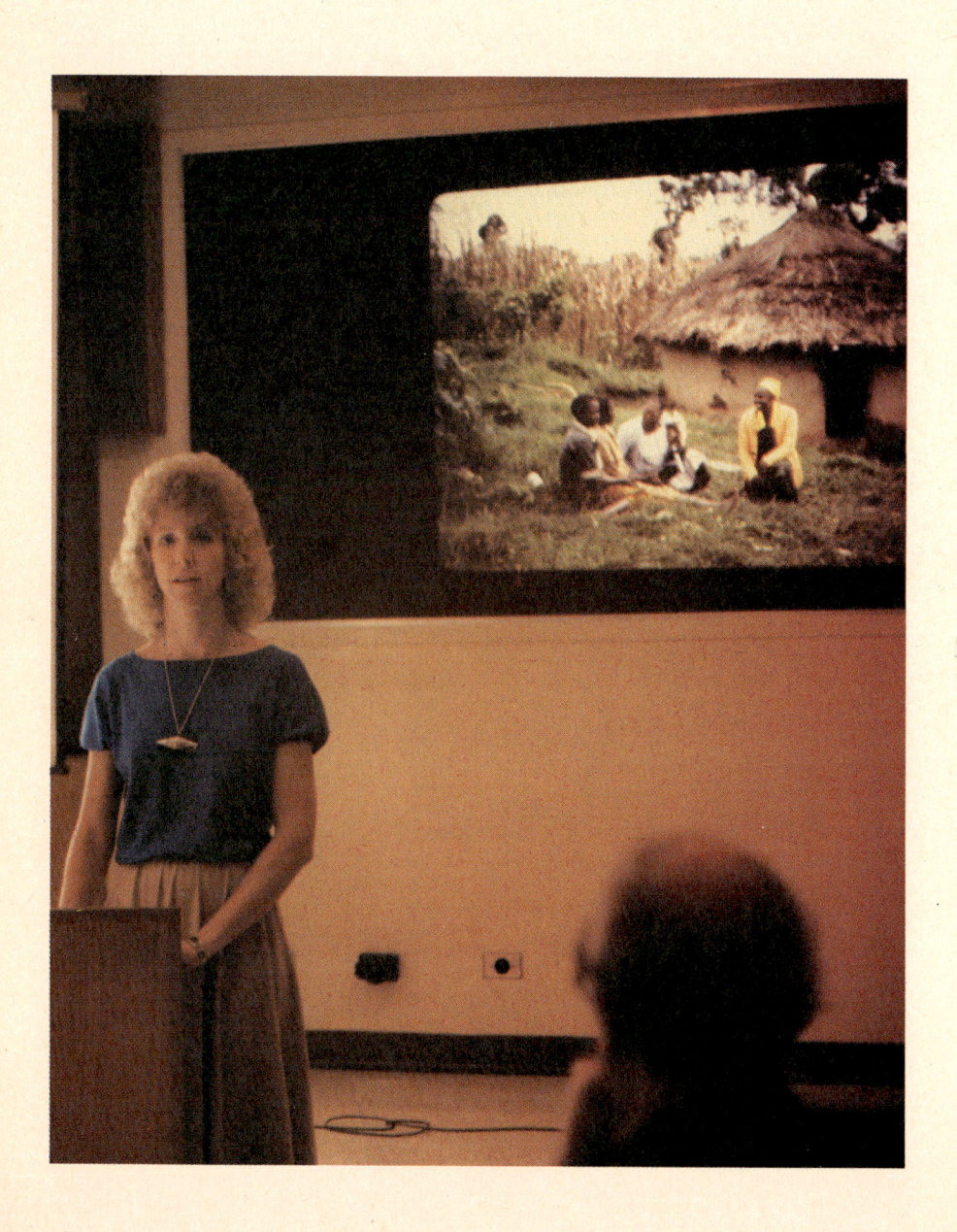

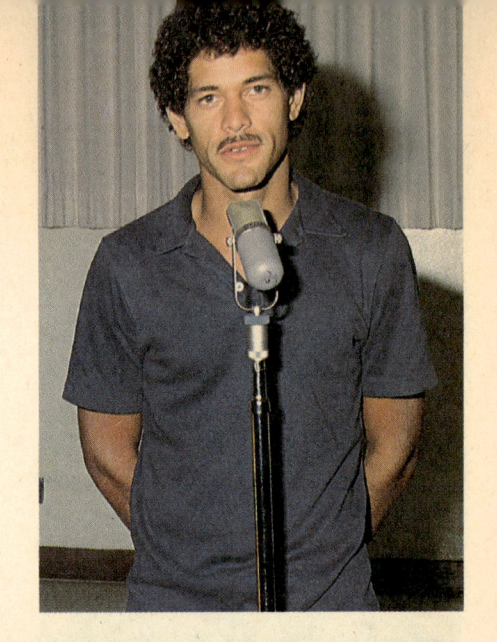

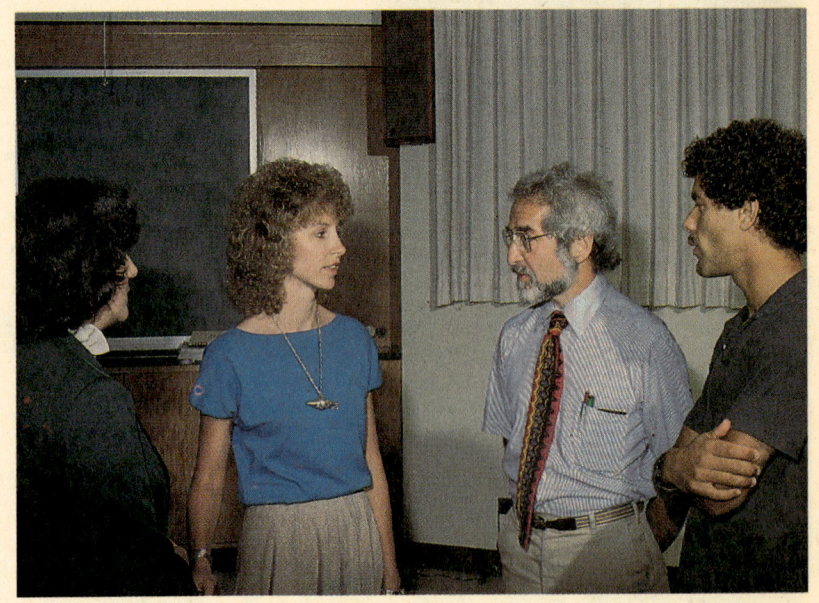

Dr. Richards gives his report next. He is investigating an illness in a rural community. He has discovered that the disease is caused by parasites, and he suspects that it is being spread through drinking water. He hopes that at the seminar he will gain insights from other doctors that can help him solve the case.

Medical detectives are often assisted by other scientists who specialize in different areas. For example, microbiologists may conduct tests with viruses and other disease-causing organisms. A microbiologist's special "suit" prevents him from being infected by the diseases with which he works.

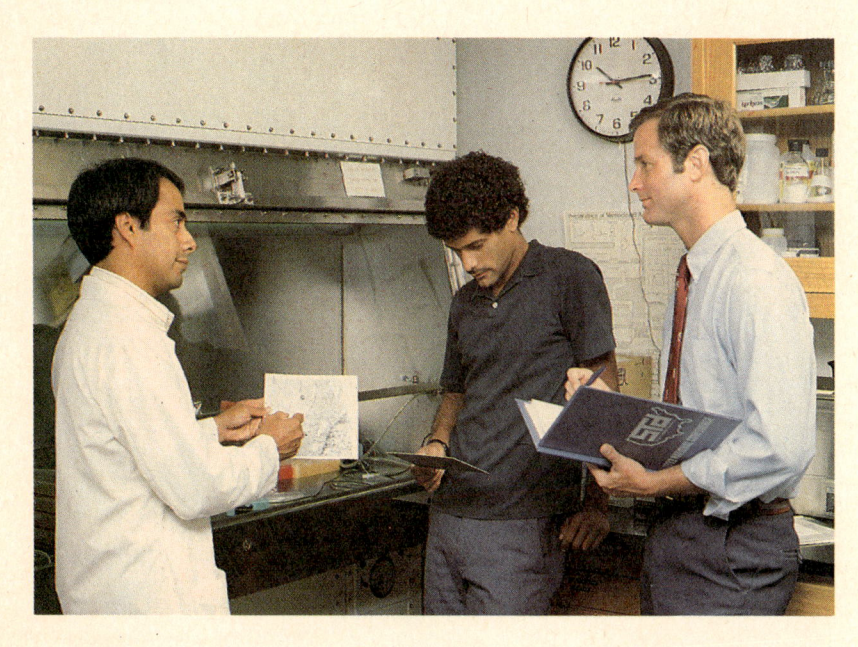

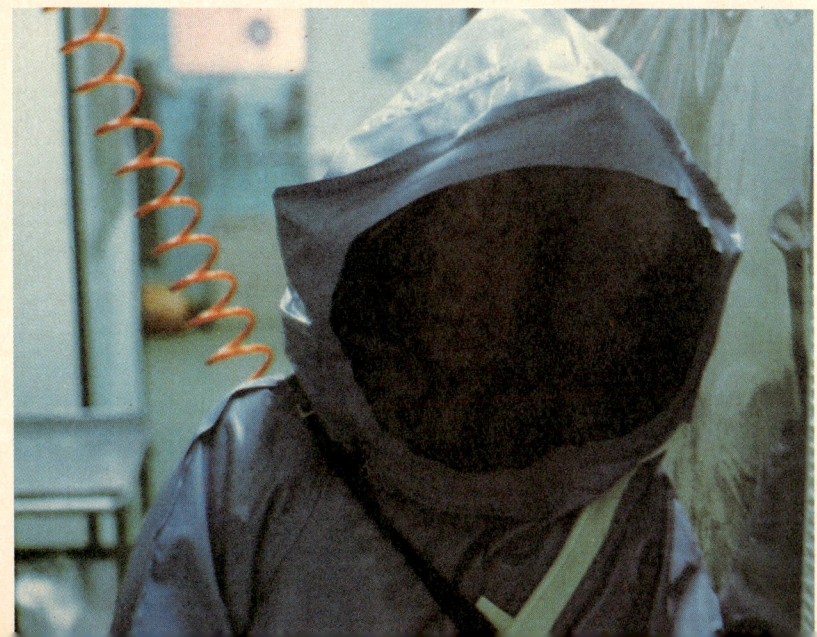

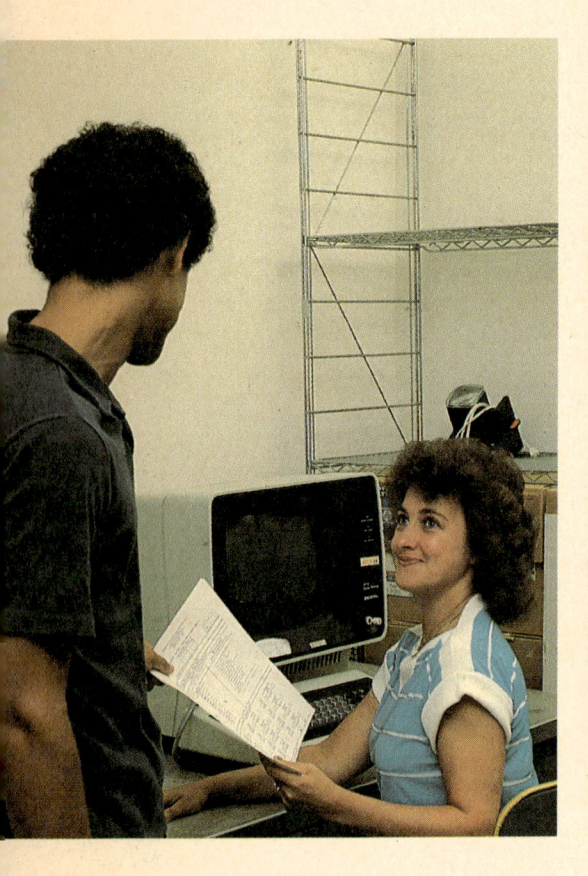

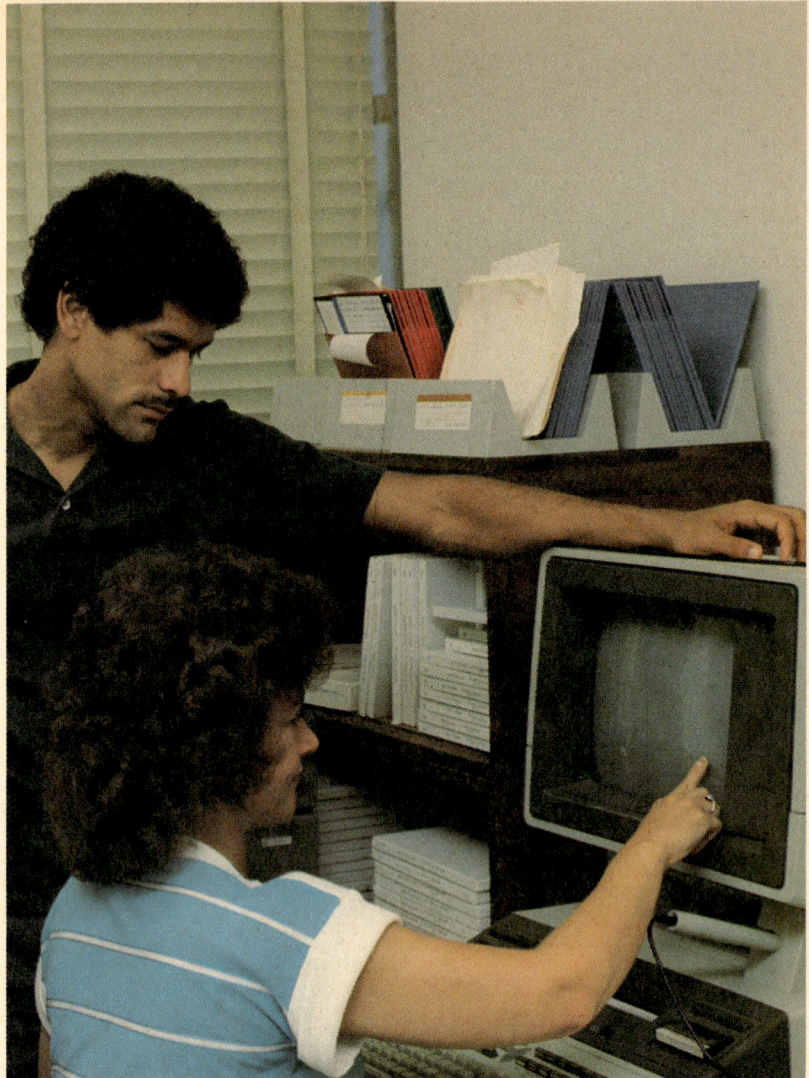

In the computer center, Dr. Richards studies graphs that show important facts related to his case—the number of patients who have the illness, and the date on which each patient became ill. He also picks up the questionnaire he will use when he interviews people in the communities where the disease has struck.

Next, he heads for the laboratory where blood samples are tested. A medical technician has just received a blood specimen, shipped to CDC's lab for analysis. While the sample is being tested, Dr. Richards discusses the case with a doctor who specializes in diseases of the blood.

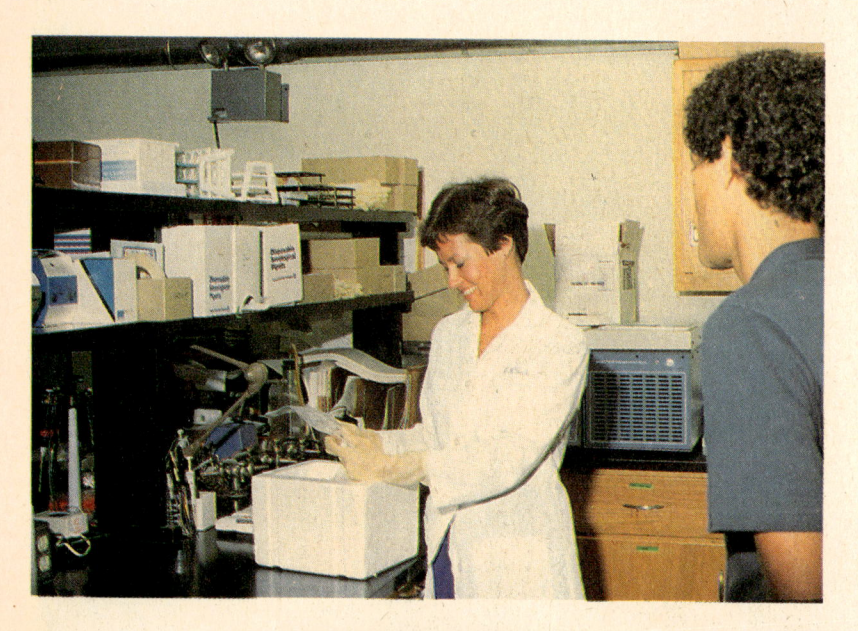

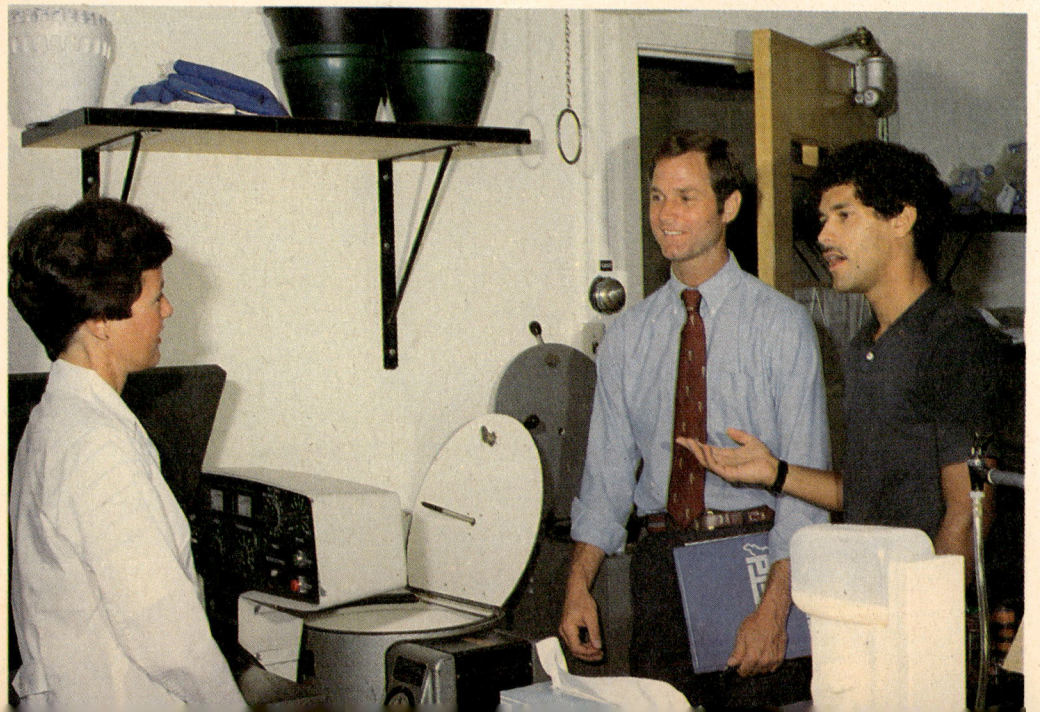

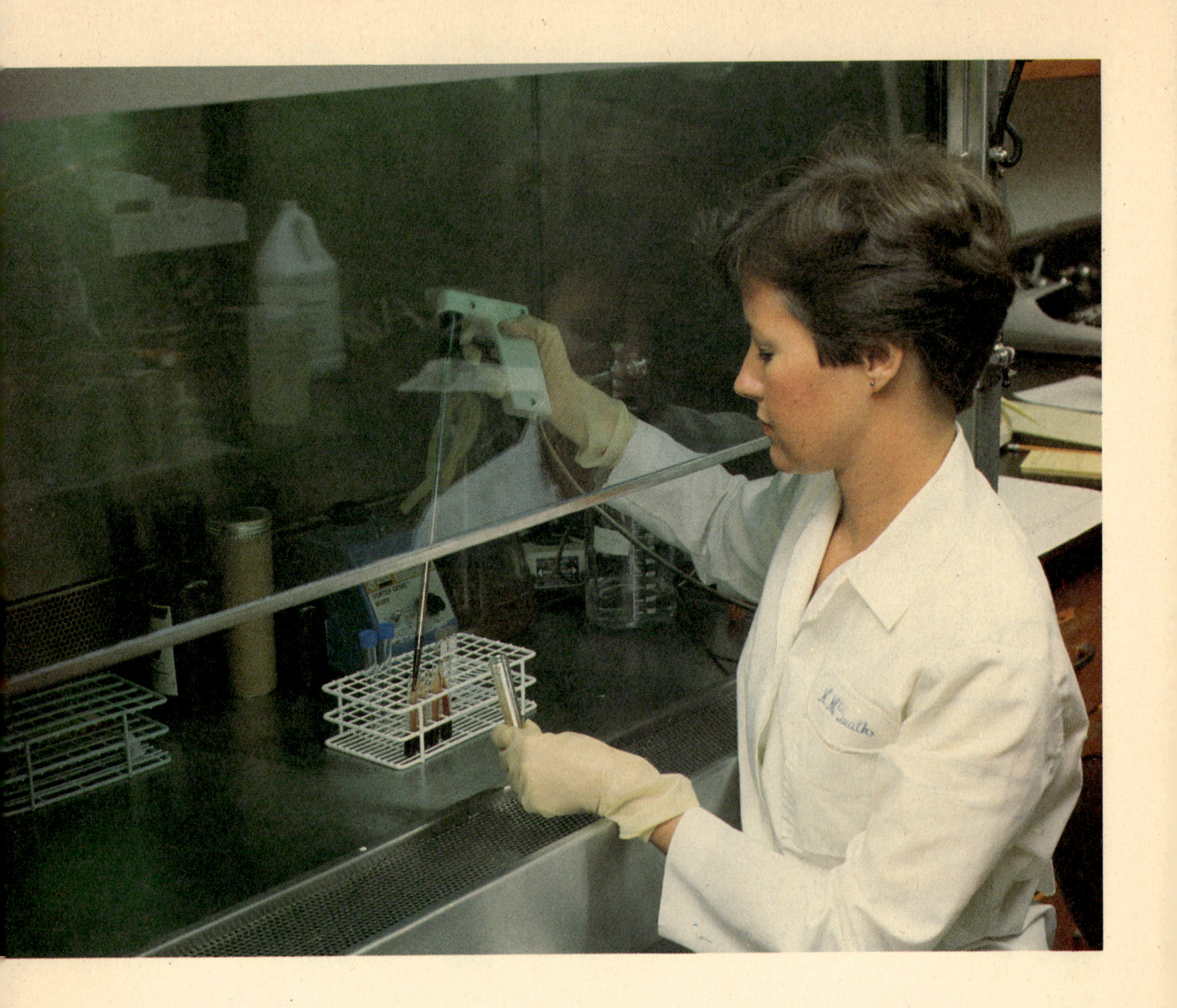

The technician divides the specimen into several parts so she can run different tests. She uses an instrument called a "pipette" to transfer the blood into several small containers. A pipette is a long, narrow glass tube that acts as a straw to withdraw and move liquids.

As the doctors continue their discussion, the technician smears a drop of blood on a thin piece of glass called a slide, and examines it under a microscope. This way she can see the individual blood cells. She knows the normal appearance of healthy blood cells. Any variations are clues that might lead to the identification of the disease.

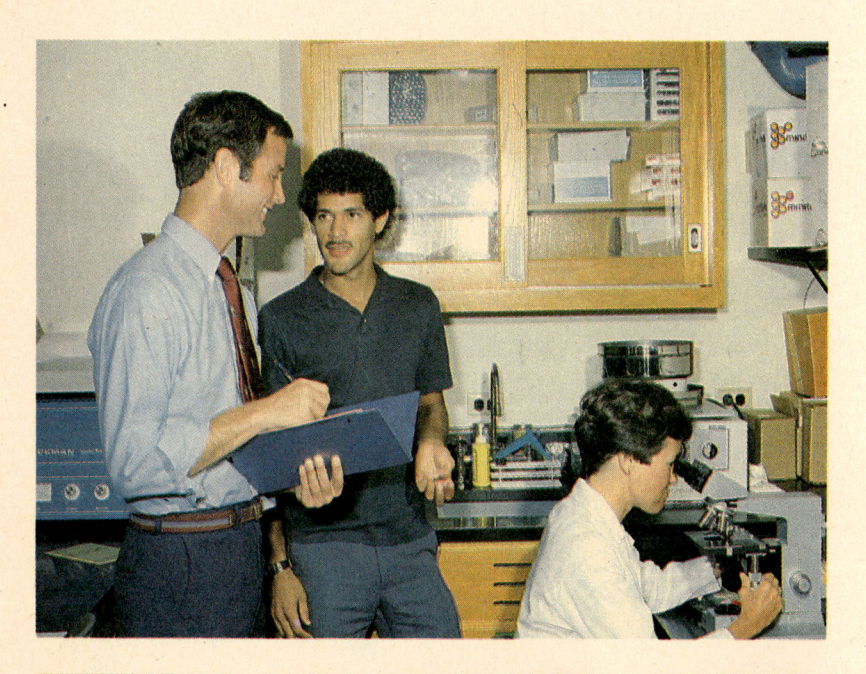

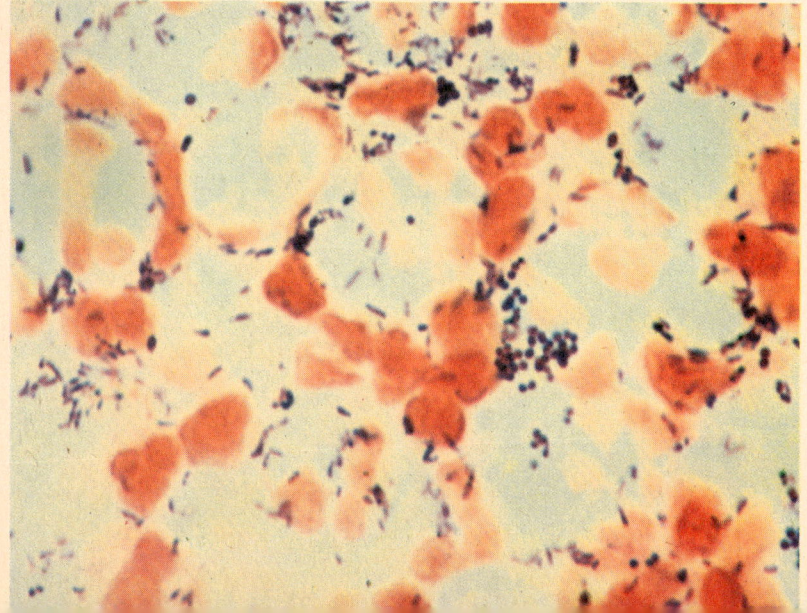

Medical detectives study all disease-causing organisms, such as parasites, viruses, and bacteria. Viruses are the hardest to detect and the most difficult to kill. But with medication, a virus can be stopped so that an infected patient will get well—and others won't get sick.

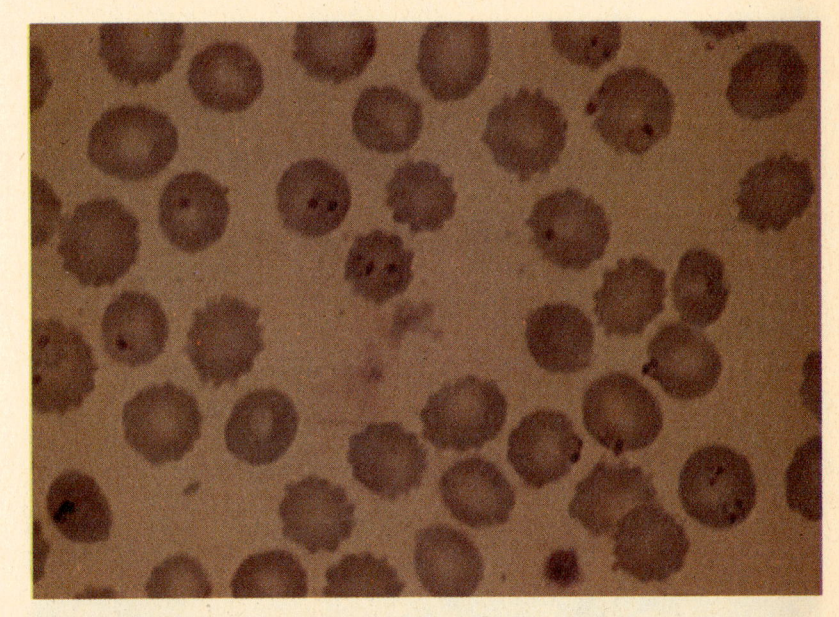

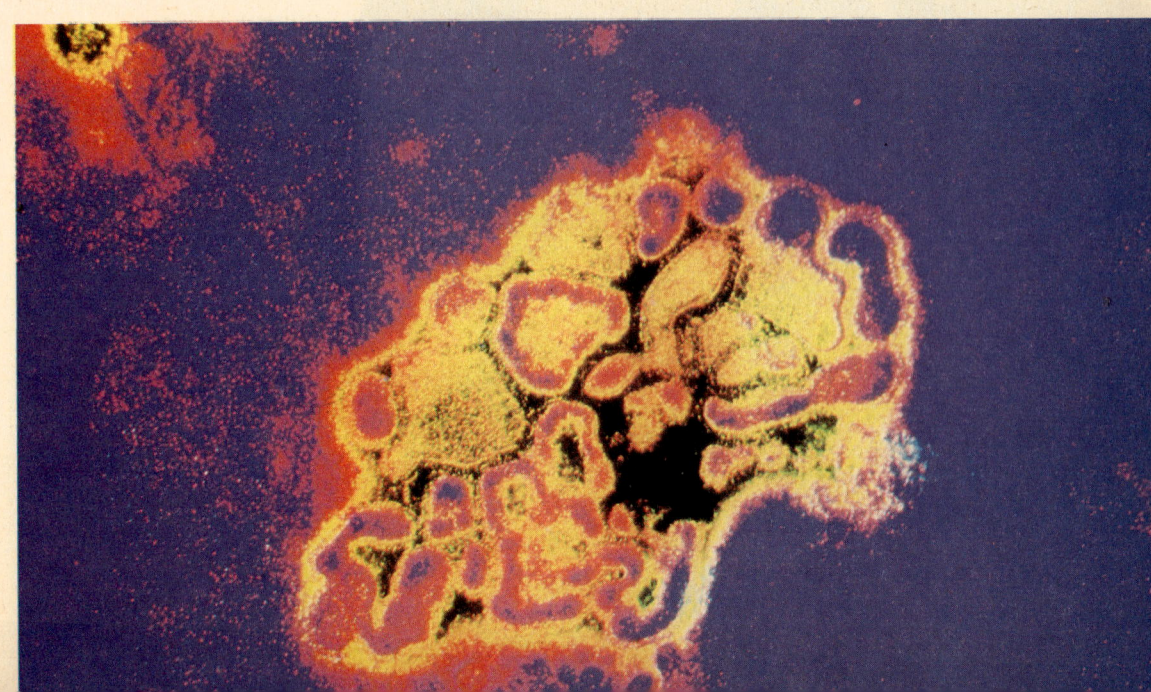

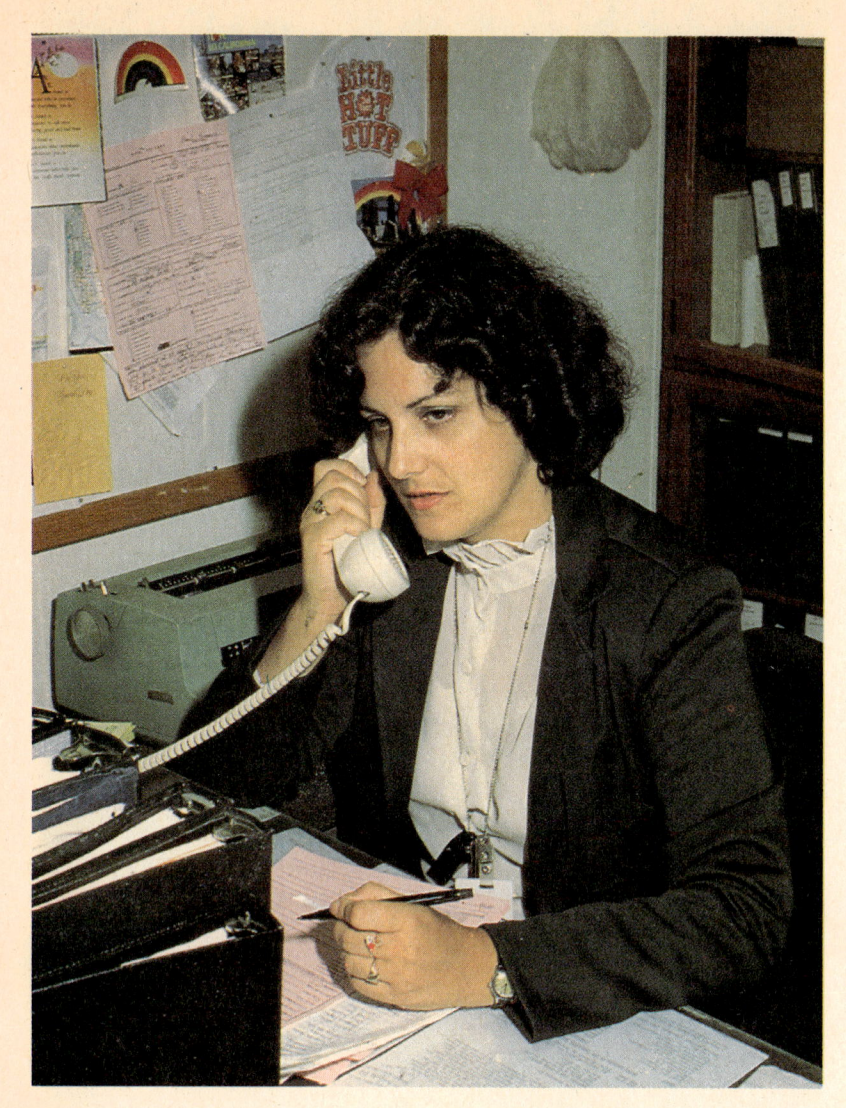

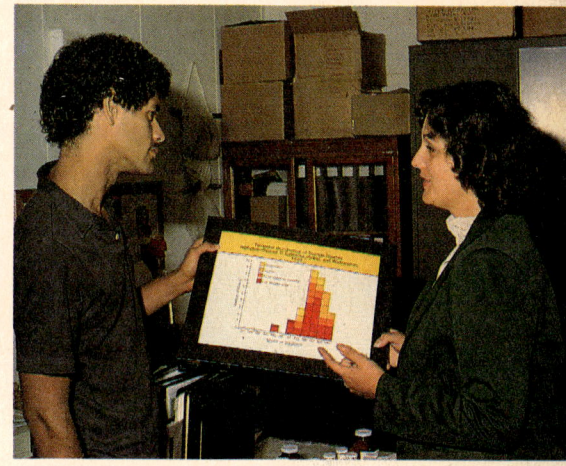

Sandy Ford is CDC's drug technician. Doctors and health officials often call her about unusual diseases. This morning, a doctor called to say that one of his patients may have eaten infected fish just before coming down with the disease Dr. Richards is investigating. Sandy shows Dr. Richards a chart illustrating a similar epidemic a few years ago.

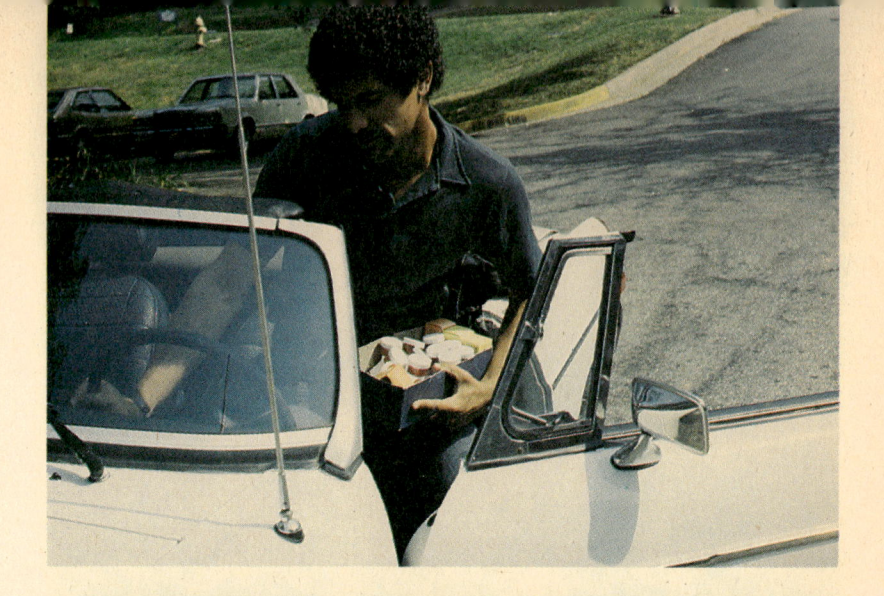

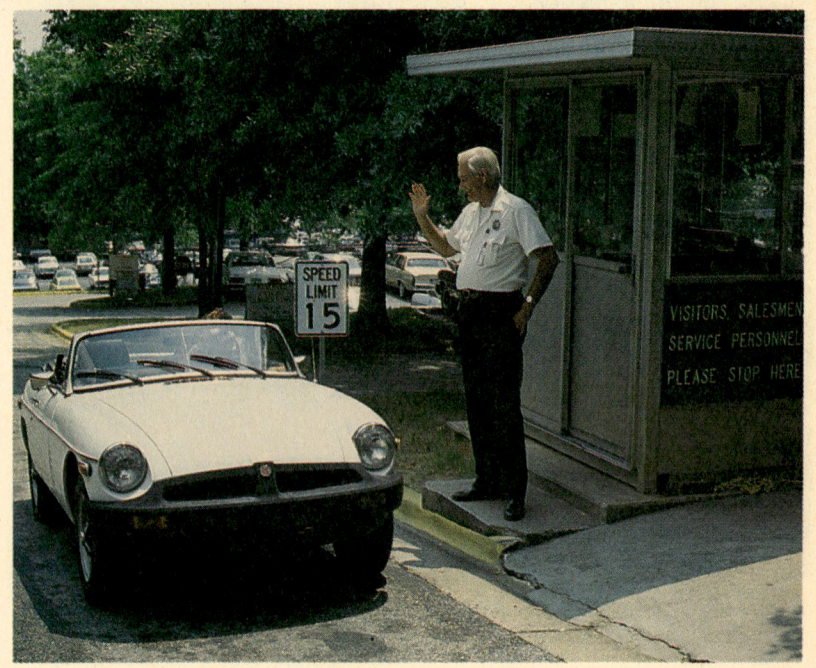

Dr. Richards puts the medicines and report forms he'll need into his car. Then he leaves CDC and drives to the area affected by the illness. He will begin his investigation by interviewing people in the area. Later he will try to piece together the information he obtains in his interviews.

As he interviews people, Dr. Richards fills out the questionnaires that were prepared at CDC. Some of the information he gets in his interviews may lead to dead ends. But some may fit into a pattern that will prove or disprove his theory that the disease is caused by a parasite in the water.

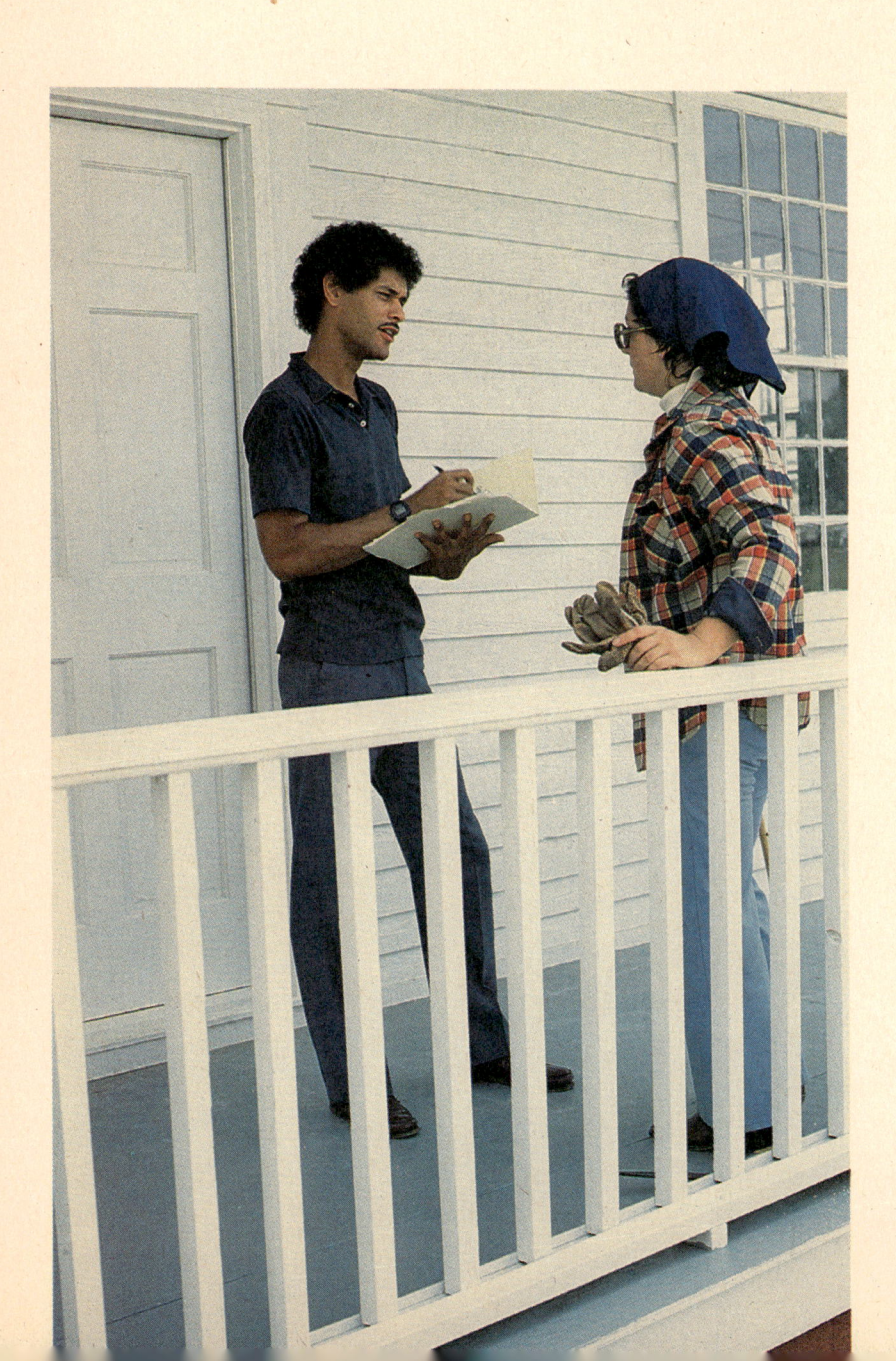

Dr. Richards visits the source of the area's water supply. Of course, there is a chance that the water could be contaminated after it leaves here, but this is the logical place to check first. He carefully looks for conditions that might indicate unhealthy water—a foul odor, rotting debris, abnormal growth of algae.

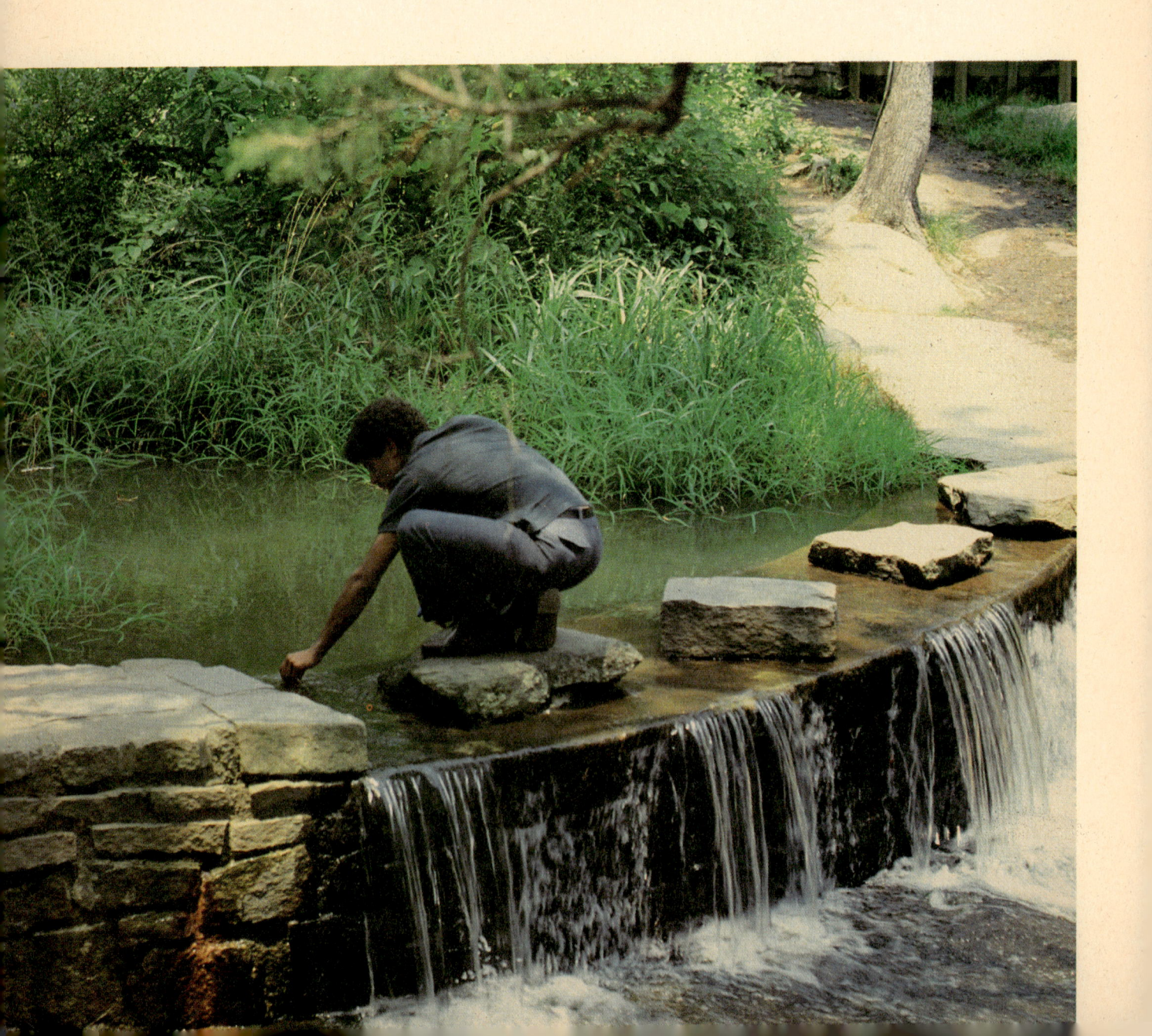

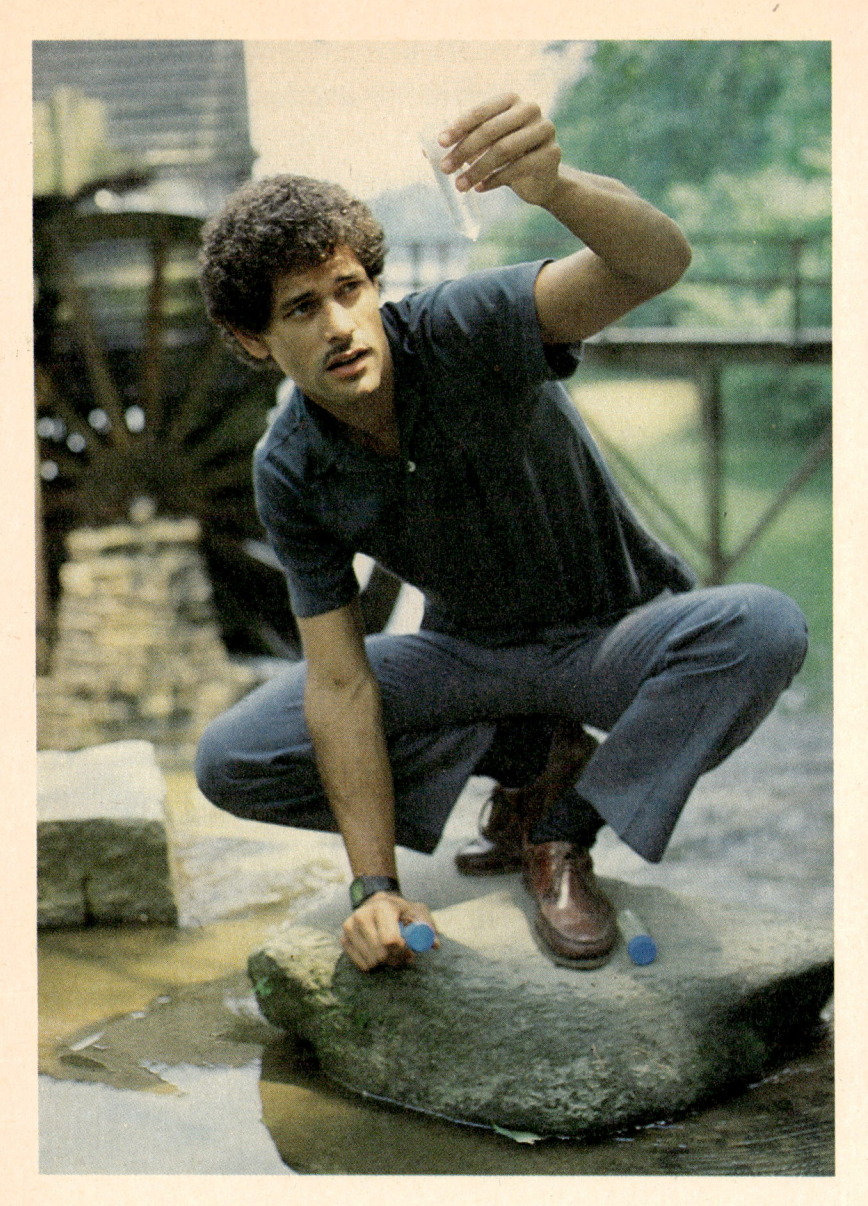

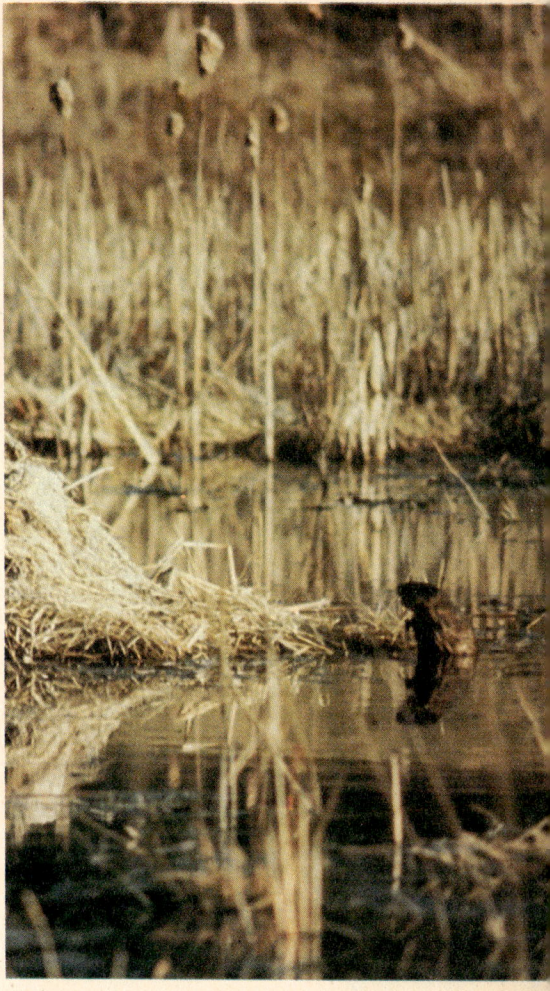

Dr. Richards takes a water sample for later analysis. Looking around the area, he spots what could turn out to be the vital missing clue. Chewed trees and beaver lodges near the watershed suggest that infected beavers may be transmitting the parasite into the water supply.

17

Working in the field, Dr. Richards wears a beeper so he can be reached if he is needed. When the beeper goes off, he locates a telephone and calls Sandy at CDC. Sandy tells him that a pilot flying from Africa to New York City has radioed a medical emergency. One of the plane's passengers was on safari in the area affected by the fever discussed at the seminar—and the passenger has taken ill.

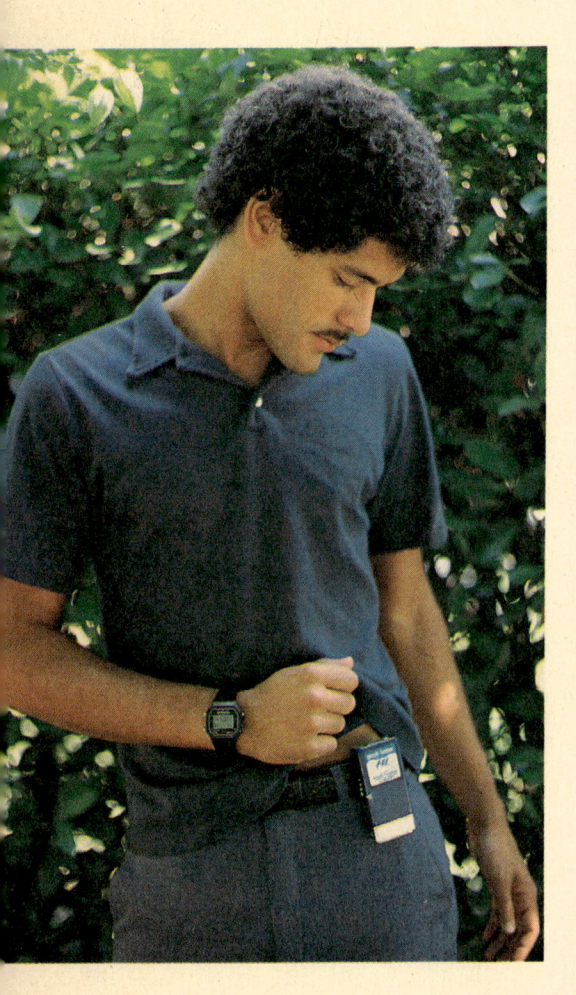

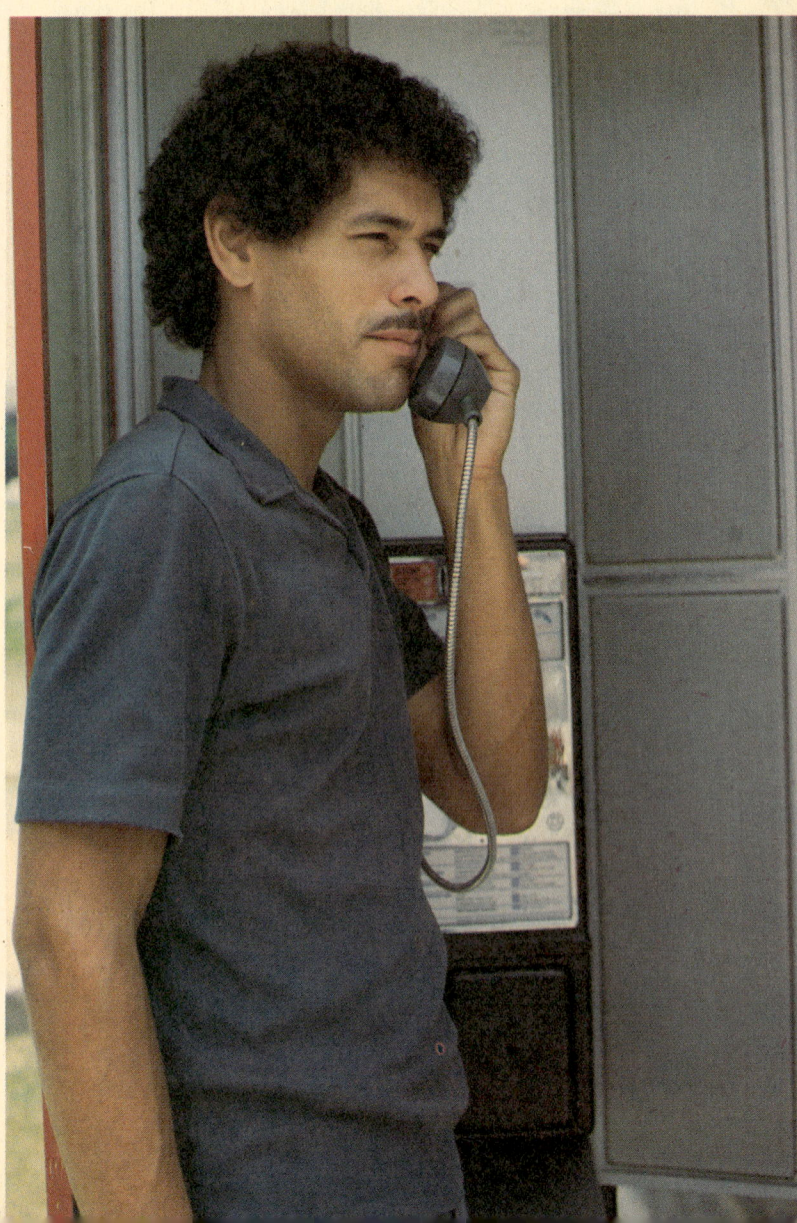

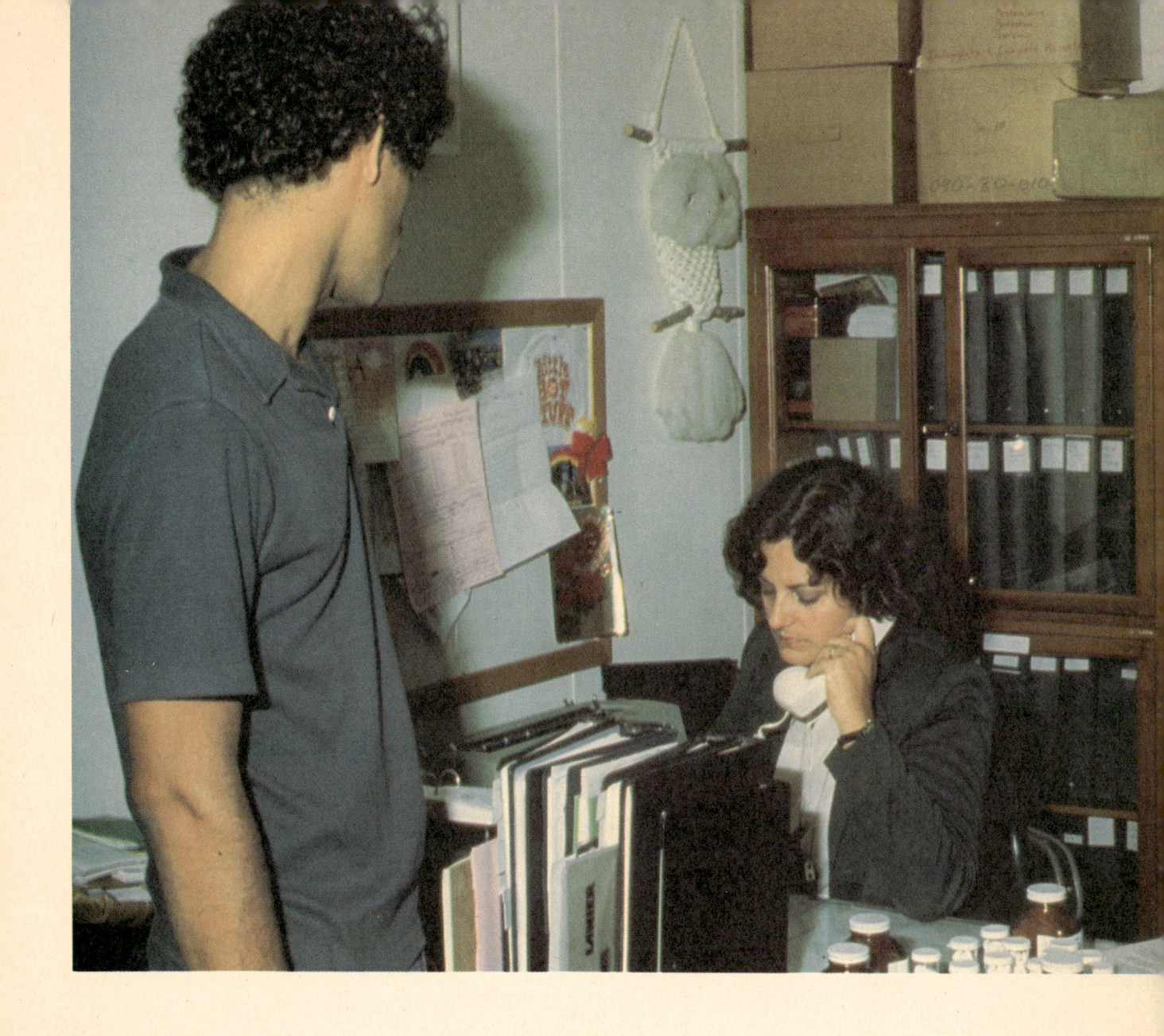

Dr. Richards returns to CDC. Sandy learns by phone that as soon as the plane lands in New York, the passenger who is ill will be rushed to the hospital. But this disease seldom occurs in the United States. The only life-saving drugs to treat it are kept at CDC, so Dr. Richards must immediately take these drugs to New York.

Dr. Richards changes his clothes, and he and Sandy pick up his ticket to New York. He has called ahead and arranged for a hospital ambulance to meet him at the airport in New York. He will be taken immediately to the hospital, where he will help administer the drugs and advise the physicians.

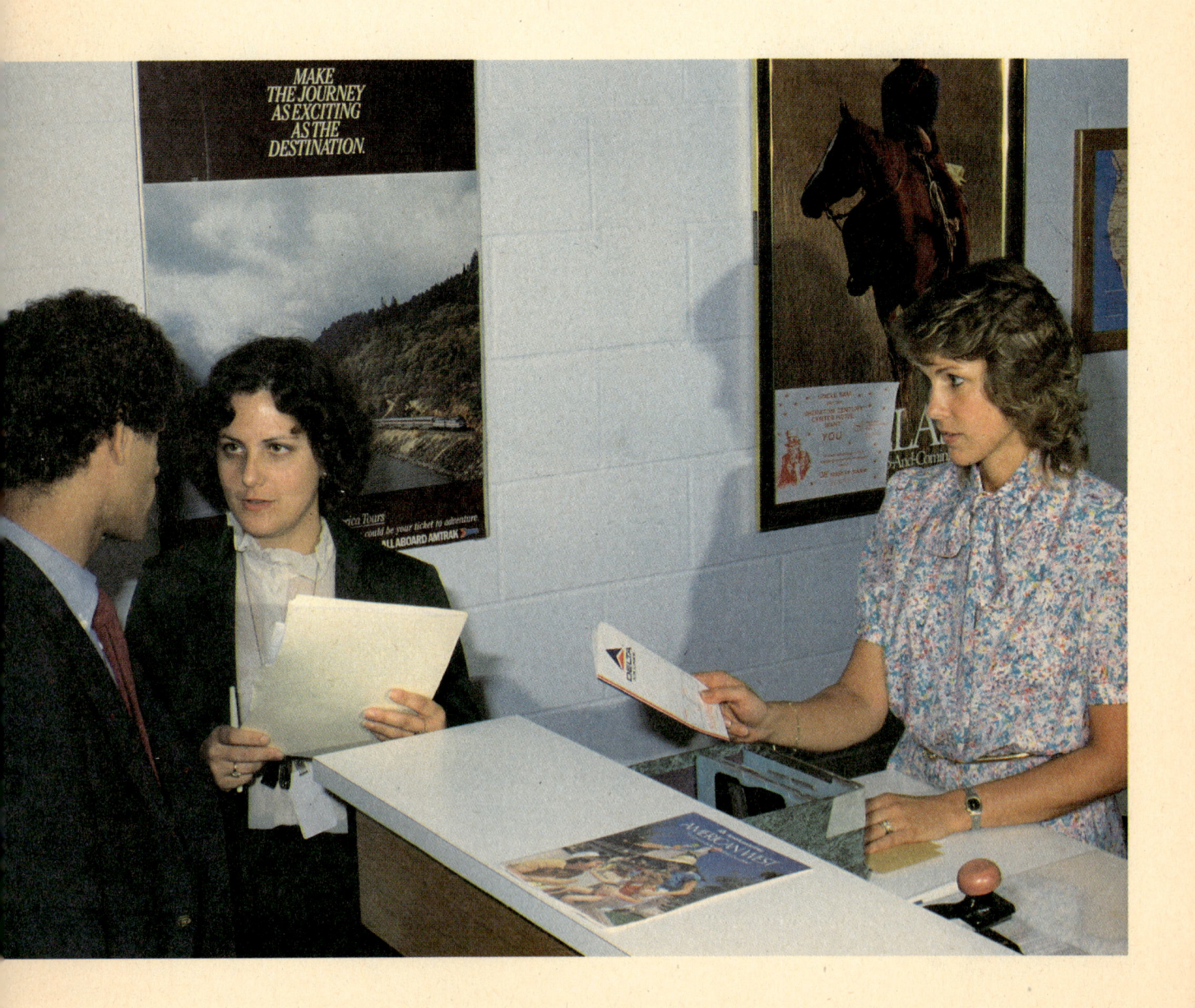

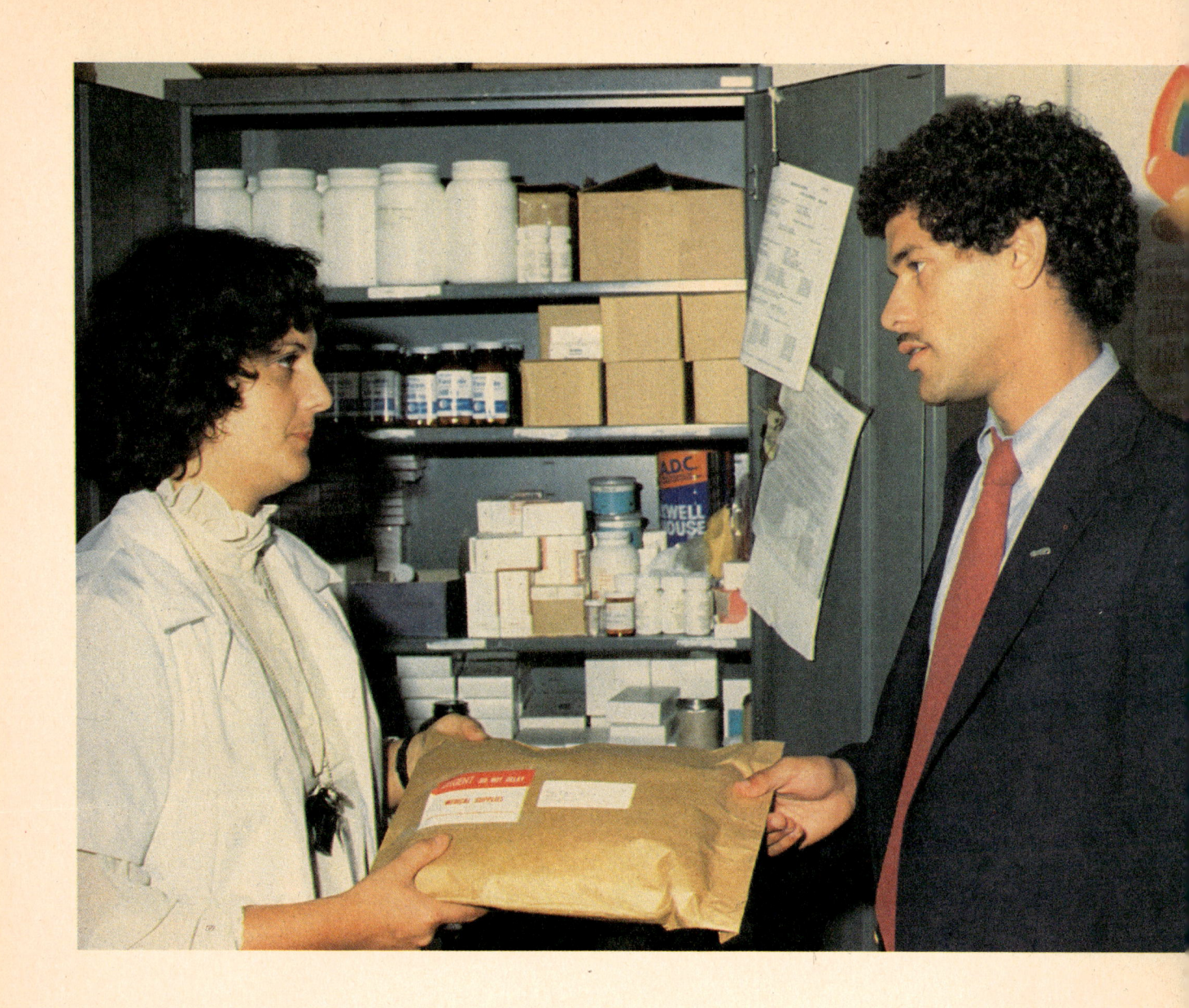

Among the medical supplies Dr. Richards will take with him are special sterile containers for specimens. He wants to bring the specimens back from New York to be analyzed by the specialists at CDC. Sandy hands him the supplies, which have been wrapped and marked "URGENT: DO NOT DELAY."

Just before he leaves for the airport, Dr. Richards hurries to the dispensary to pick up the special medicines that he must deliver to New York. They must be kept frozen, so they are placed in an insulated container and marked "PERISHABLE. KEEP FROZEN." As soon as the medicine is packed, Dr. Richards is on his way.

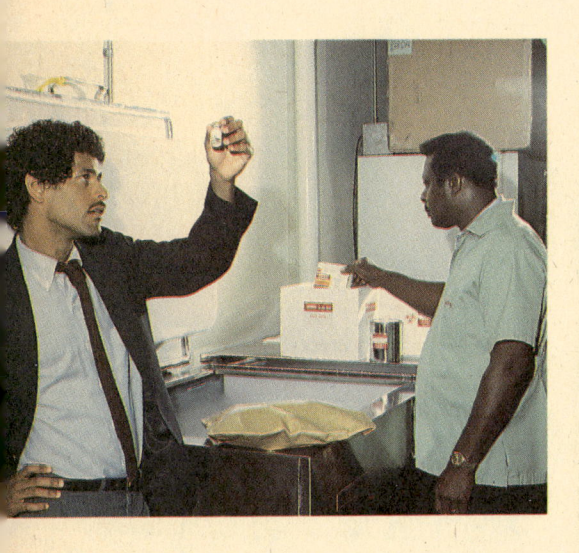

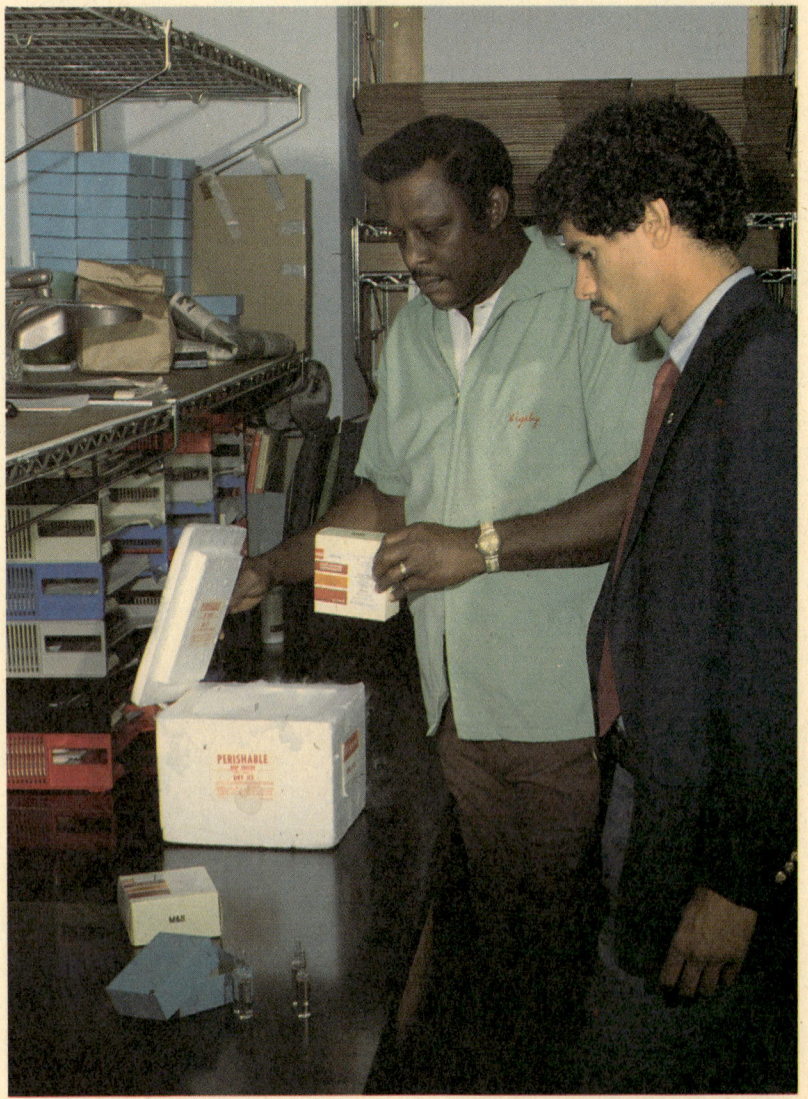

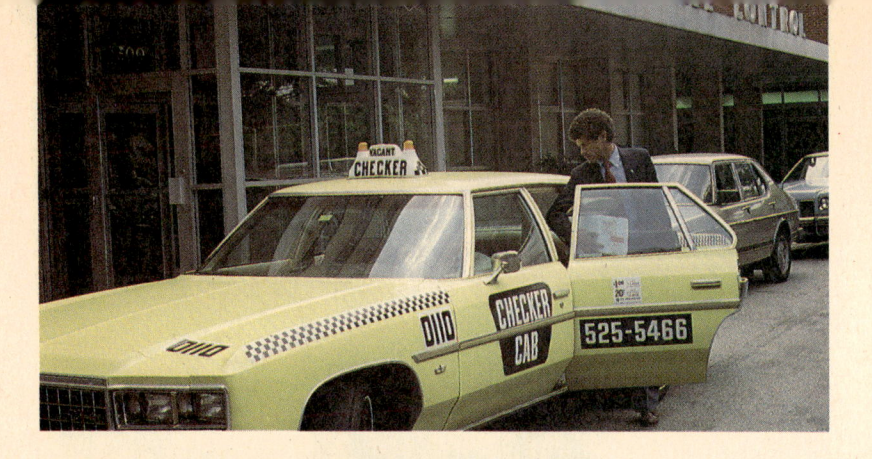

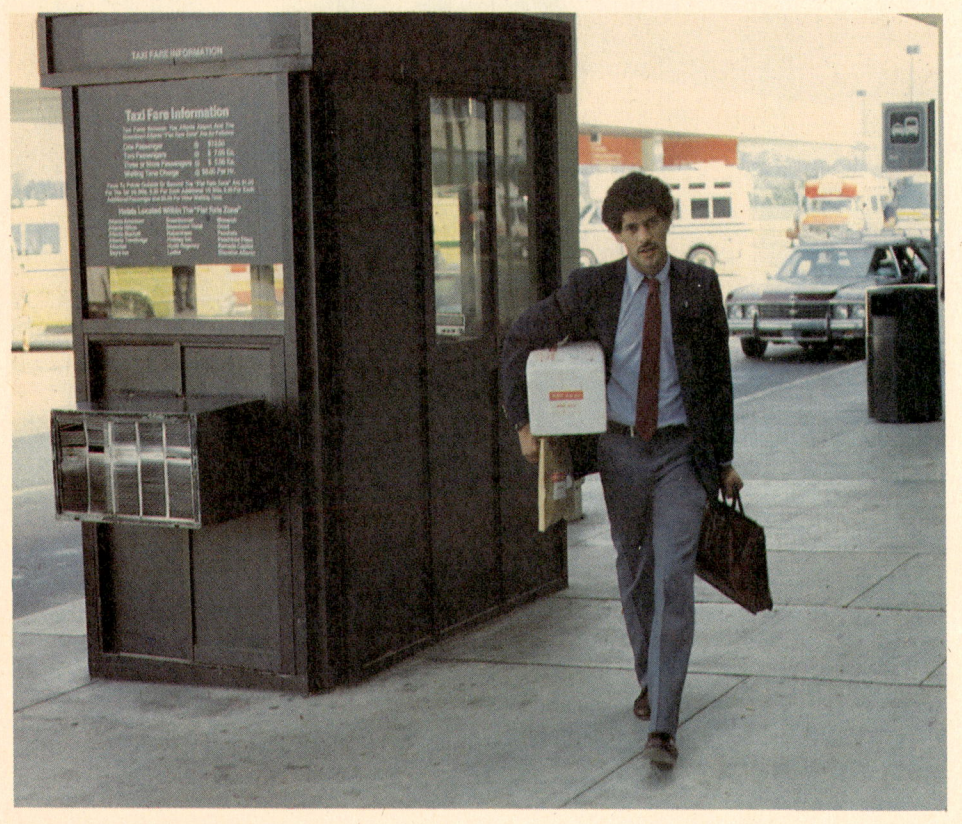

A taxi takes him to the airport. All he carries with him are the emergency medications, medical supplies, and a briefcase. When he arrives at the airport, he goes straight inside. The airline has been informed of the medical emergency, and is expecting him.

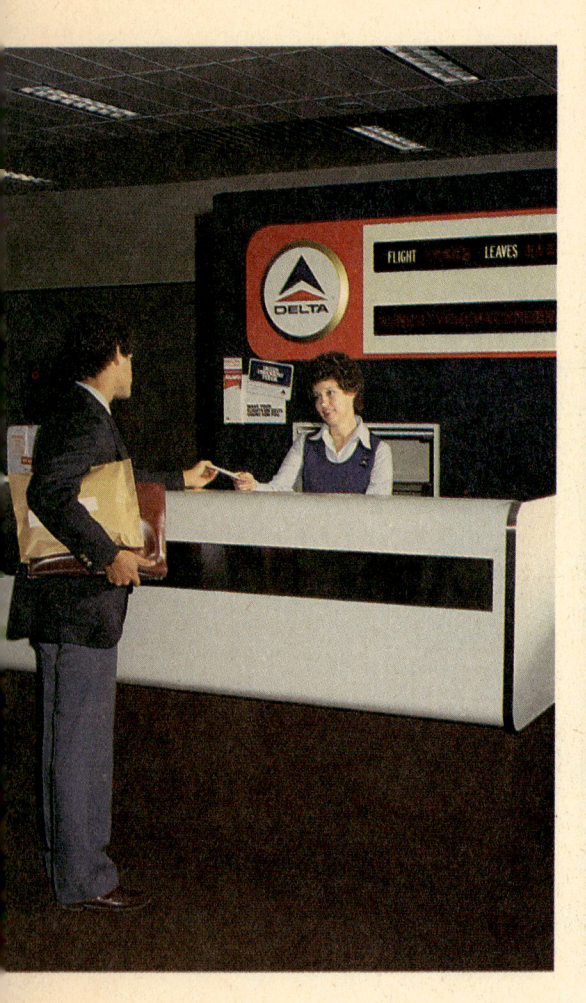

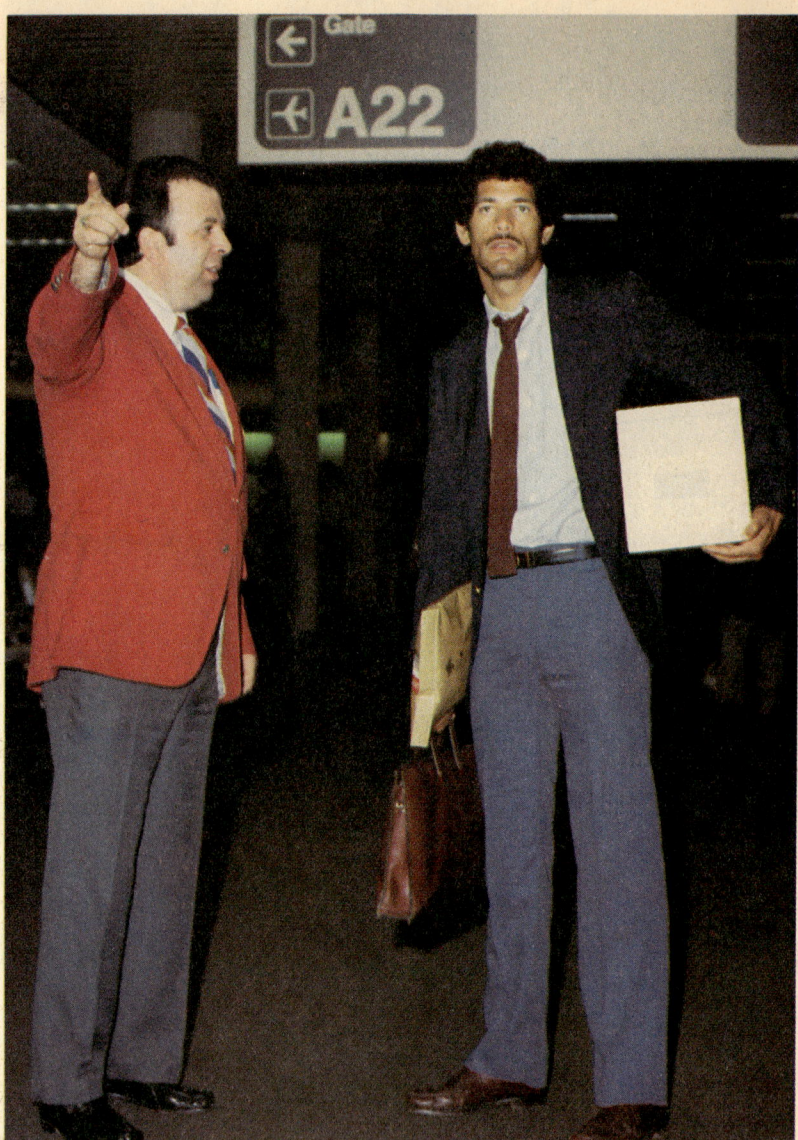

The airline attendant knows that Dr. Richards is traveling in an official capacity for CDC. She quickly takes his ticket and hands him his boarding pass. Then an airline official points out the gate where the plane is waiting for Dr. Richards to board.

Aboard the plane, the flight attendant tells him that he will be the first passenger to leave the plane when they arrive in New York. Then Dr. Richards gets down to work. He must review medical literature on each illness he thinks could be affecting the traveler. Then he will note the laboratory tests he'll want done, and list the additional drugs he may need.

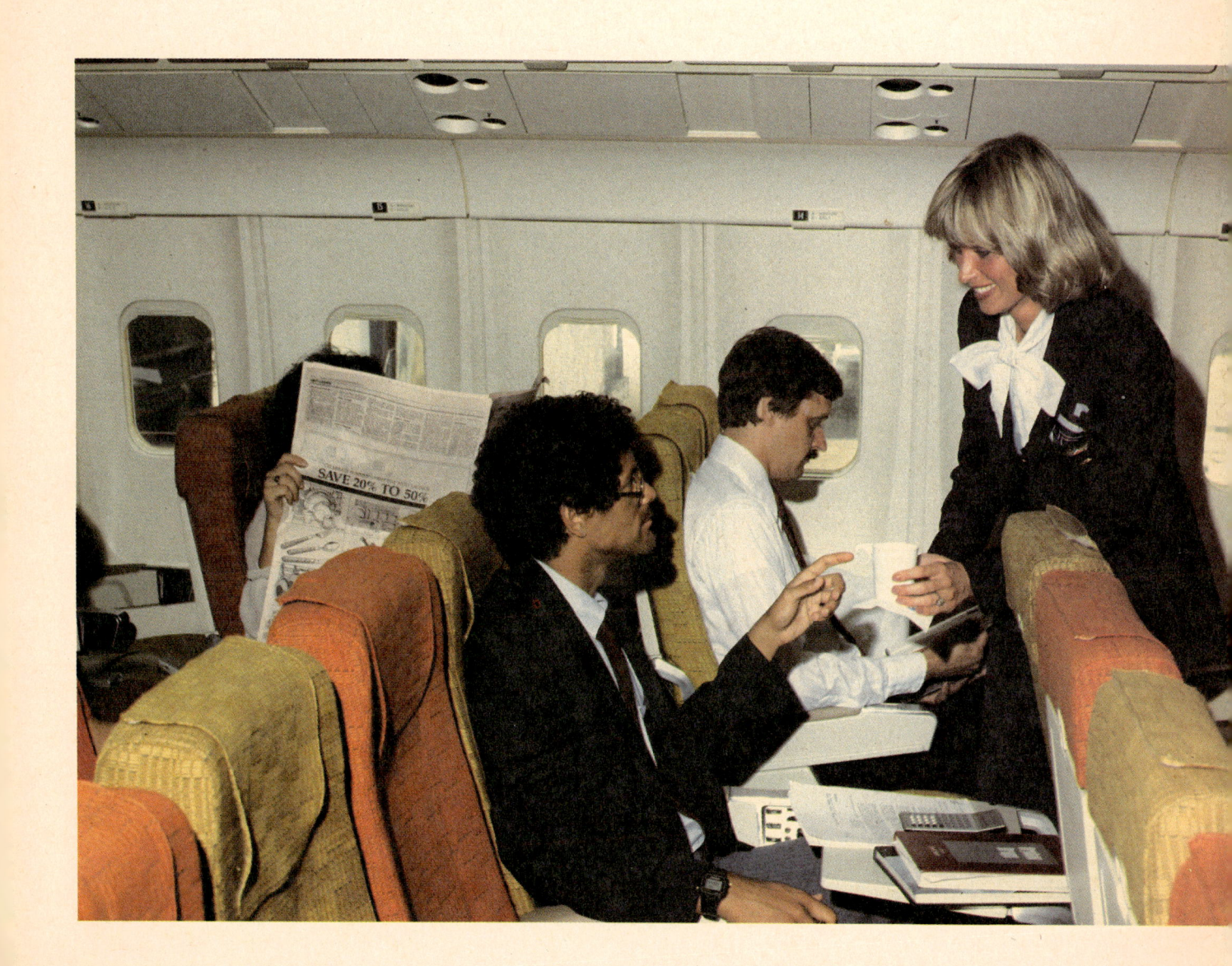

When Dr. Richards lands in New York, the quarantine officer who inspected the plane from Africa greets him. The officer provides him with as much information about the case as he can. As Dr. Richards gets into the waiting ambulance, the attendants radio the hospital to let the doctors know that the medicine is on its way.

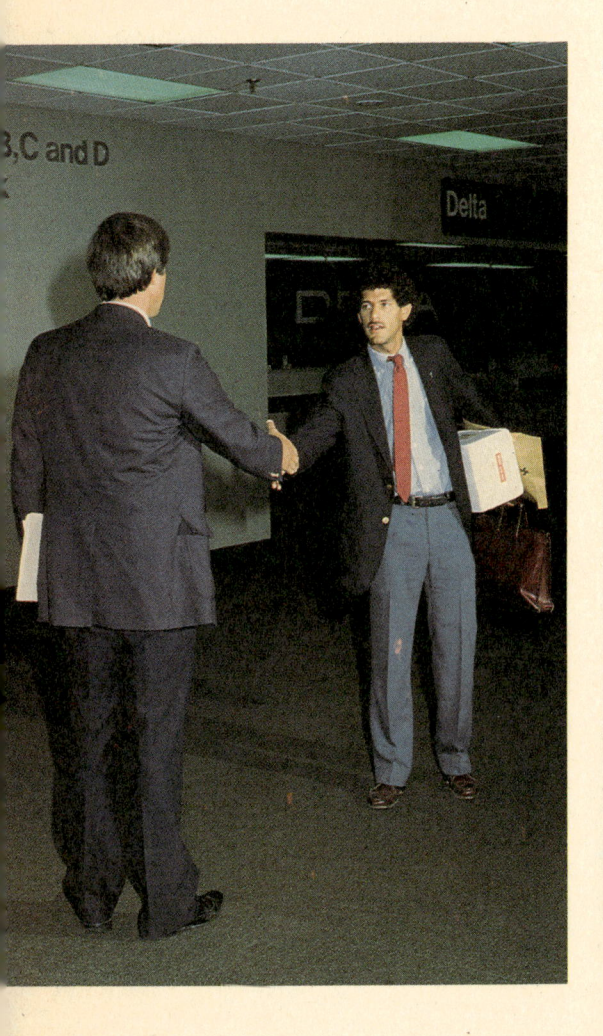

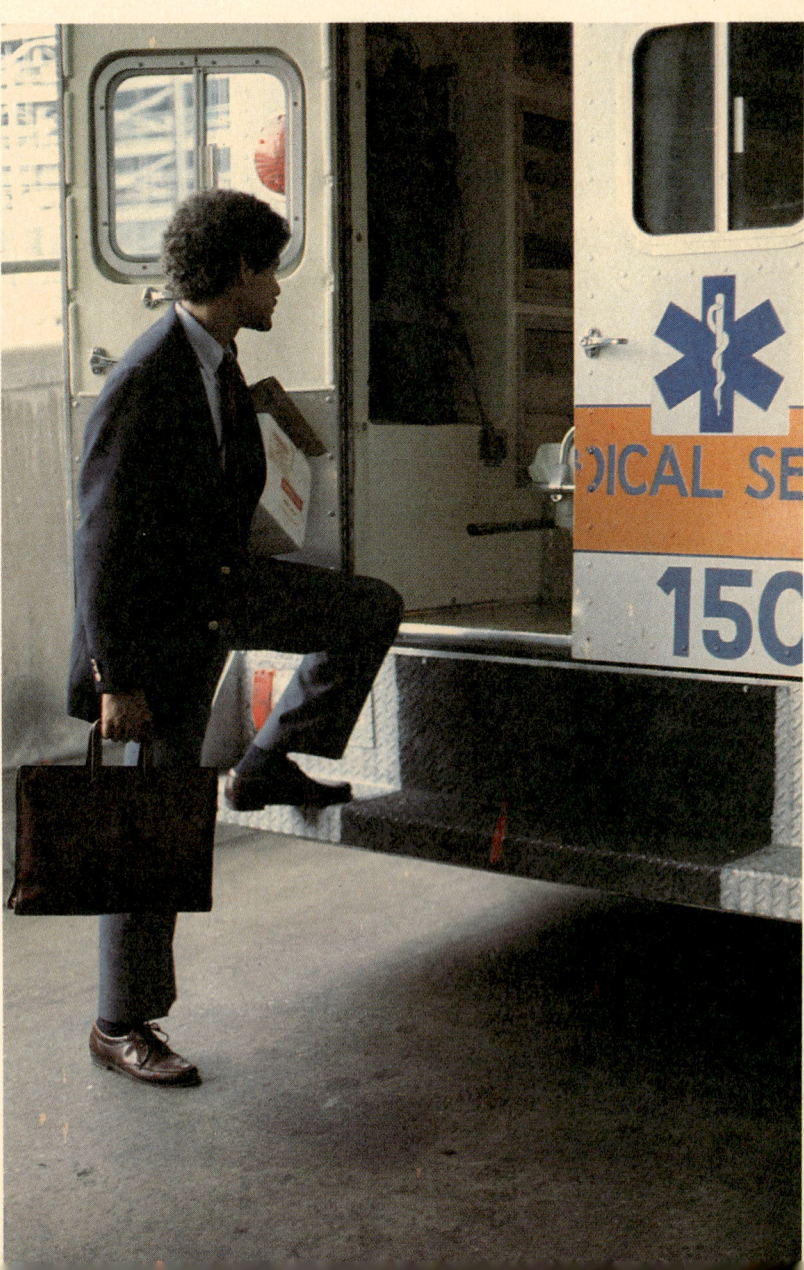

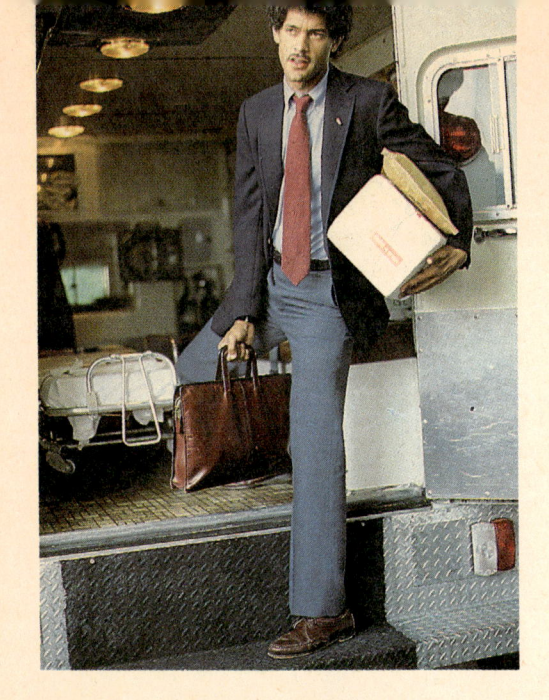

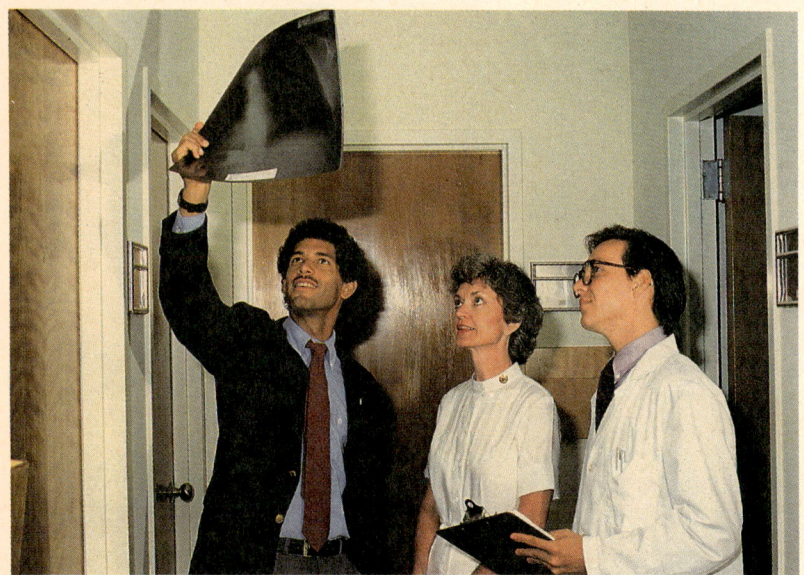

Dr. Richards arrives at the hospital and hurries inside. He meets with the doctors involved with the case, and together they review the patient's x-rays and discuss his symptoms. It is important to determine exactly what is causing the illness as soon as possible, so that treatment can begin.

27

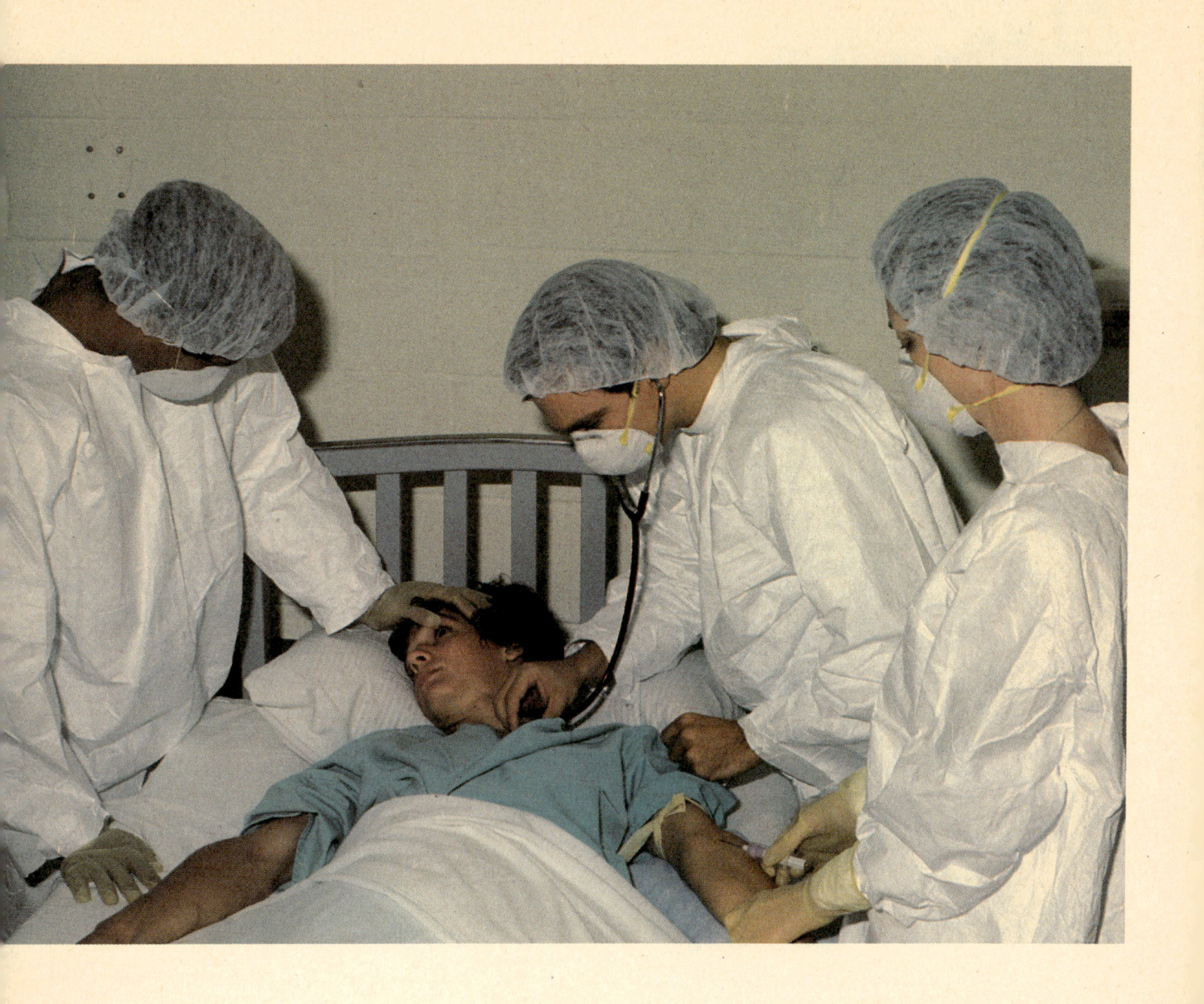

Several tests have been performed, but the doctors are still not positive about the cause of the disease. Putting on a sterile gown and mask for protection, Dr. Richards joins the doctors who are examining the patient. He checks the heartbeat, takes blood samples, and conducts a thorough physical examination.

Finally the medical team identifies the cause of the disease. It is the parasite responsible for African sleeping sickness. Now the treatment can begin. Dr. Richards carefully measures the special medicine he has brought from CDC. The life-saving medicine will be injected with a hypodermic needle.

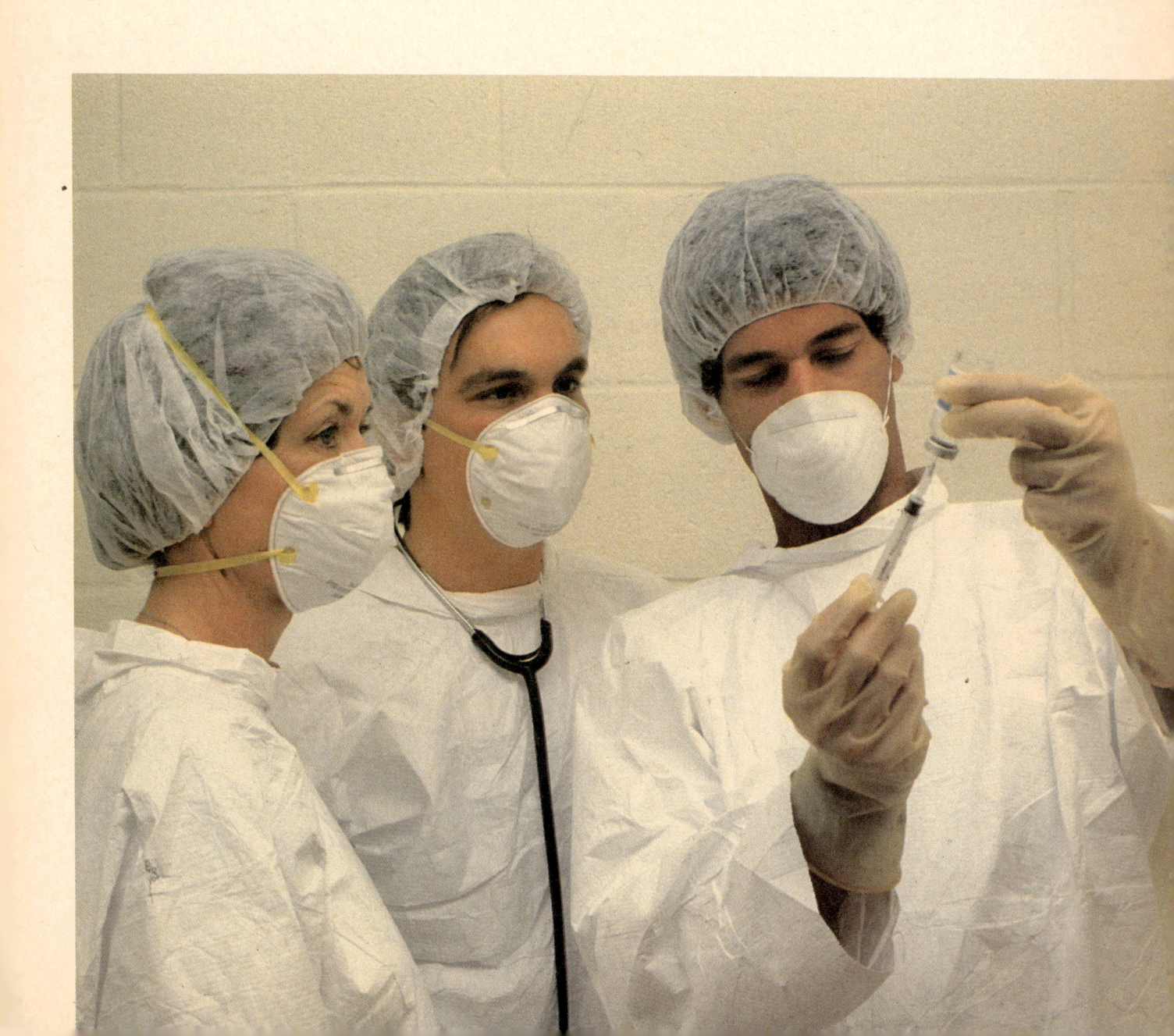

It is particularly important to give exactly the right amount of medicine. Giving a patient too little will not kill the parasite, and the patient's condition may worsen. Giving too much can also be dangerous. After Dr. Richards prepares the hypodermic, one of the hospital's physicians injects it into the patient's arm.

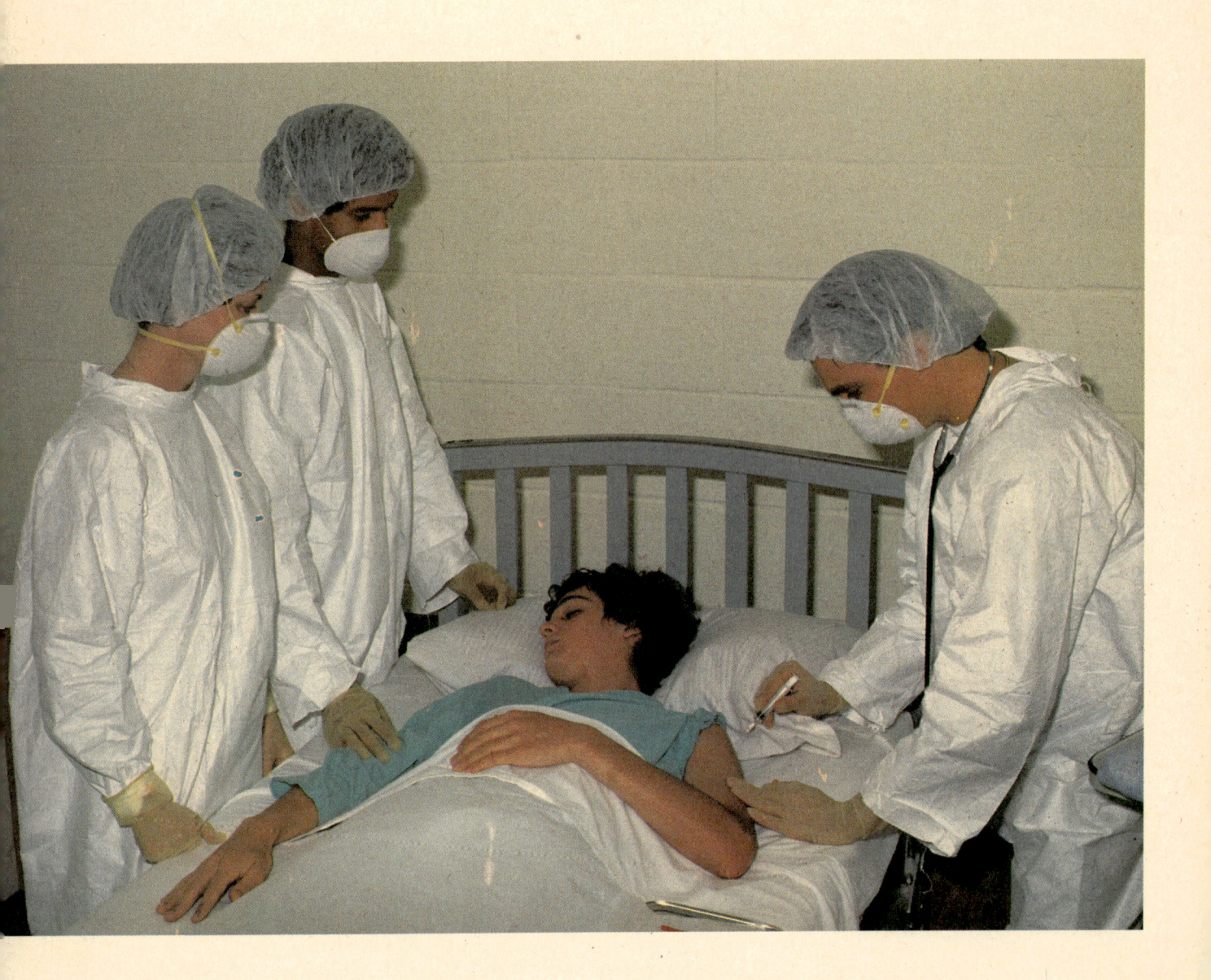

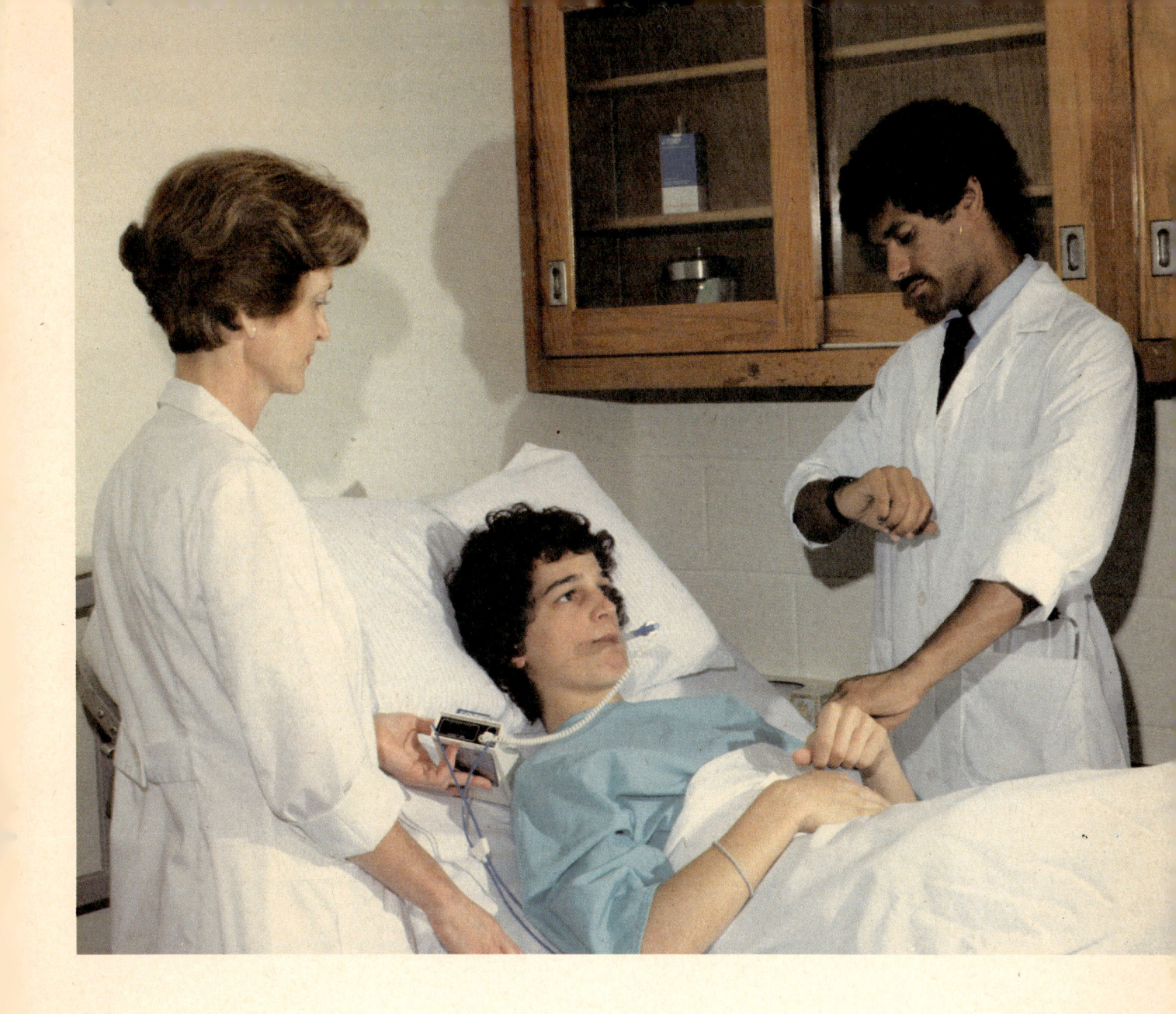

Within hours after the drug is injected, the patient should be visibly better. Within a few days, recovery should be complete. There should be no permanent damage, because treatment was begun in time. Dr. Richards will monitor the patient's condition for several hours before leaving the hospital.

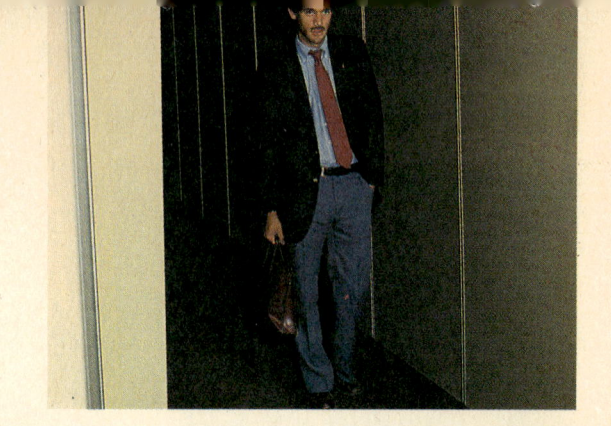

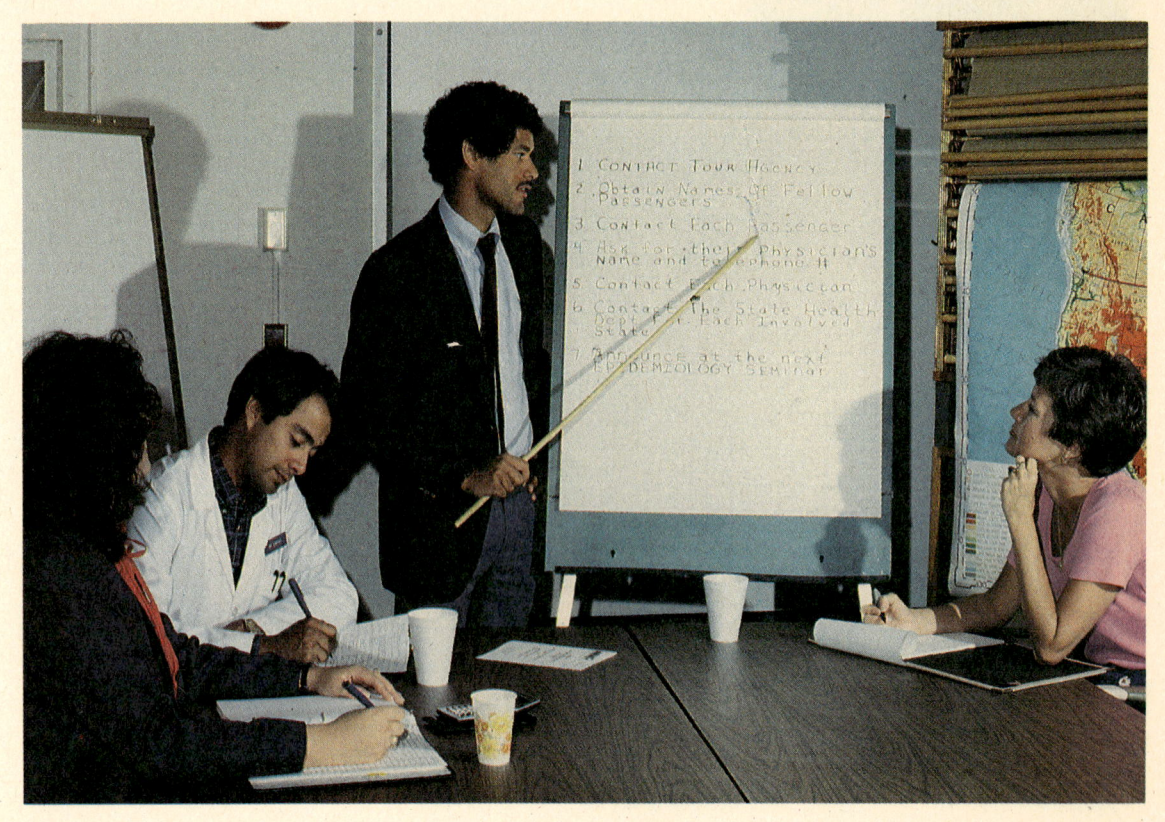

Dr. Richards catches the 5:30 a.m. flight back to Atlanta. At CDC, he briefs his coworkers, who will contact the other passengers and alert them to early signs of the infection. Some workdays—like the past 24 hours—are longer and more hectic than others. But Dr. Richards is used to that. For a medical detective, it's all part of the job.